C
in

One Foot in the Stars

THE STORY OF AN
EXTRAORDINARY
HEALER

MATTHEW MANNING
AND TESSA ROSE

PIATKUS

Copyright © 2003 by Matthew Manning and Tessa Rose

First published by Element in 1999

This edition first published in 2003 by
Judy Piatkus (Publishers) Limited
5 Windmill Street
London W1T 2JA
e-mail: info@piatkus.co.uk

The moral right of the author has been asserted

A catalogue record for this book is available from the British Library

ISBN 0 7499 2463 2

Edited by Krystyna Mayer
Text design by Jerry Goldie

This book has been printed on paper manufactured
with respect for the environment using wood from managed
sustainable resources

Typeset by Palimpsest Book Production Limited,
Polmont, Stirlingshire
Printed and bound in Great Britain by
Bookmarque Ltd, Croydon, Surrey

OTHER BOOKS BY MATTHEW MANNING:

The Link
In the Minds of Millions
Strangers
Matthew Manning's Guide to Self-healing
No Faith Required
The Healing Journey

CONTENTS

For Gig, Henrietta and Jethro –
Now you know the whole story!

Preface

In interviews and during my seminars, the question that I am most frequently asked is, 'How did you become a healer?' It's a story that began over thirty-five years ago, and which has continued right through to the present day. To give a quick or succinct answer is therefore never easy! As the interviewers and seminar participants get younger, I realise that many of them were either very young – or possibly not yet born – when I first came to the attention of the public in the early 1970s.

By many people's standards I have had an extraordinary life in which I've had to learn to live with a gift that – for whatever reason – was bestowed upon me. I have always tried to use this gift to help as many others as possible, but it has also taught me a great deal about both others and myself over the decades. Healing has long been shrouded in mystery and regarded with scepticism and suspicion, but I like to think that I have helped the subject to become more widely accepted and 'mainstream'.

I am not a spiritual leader or writer, but I know that my work has attracted the interest of thousands of people who, like me, are looking for 'something else' in life without the dogma of religion. As I move through middle age, I am aware that I've now got more decades behind me than in front of me. I'm not sufficiently vain to believe that I will be remembered long after I've gone, but I sometimes like to think that perhaps one day someone will find *One Foot in the Stars* in a second-hand bookshop and learn a little bit more about healing and one man who made it his life.

Matthew Manning, 2003

Chapter 1

ONE FOOT IN
THE STARS

My earliest memory is of sitting in a high-chair in a light-filled room with sliding glass windows. I am being fed by my mother and refusing to eat the food because she has told me it is chicken. I can remember thinking it was cruel to eat chicken. I am not a vegetarian.

I should not be surprised if this was one of the early instances that led to my mother branding me 'as obstinate as a cartload of monkeys'. If I was set on doing something nothing could stop me, and if I did not want to do something, nothing could make me. I could not be shifted one way or the other.

Paradoxically, I was also paralysed by shyness. My mother says that I was so shy that if anyone I did not know called at the house I would hide behind or under the furniture. I do not think anyone can appreciate how difficult shyness is to cope with unless they have been shy themselves. I will always remember my first day at primary school. I was desperate to go to the loo but was too shy and too embarrassed to put my hand up to ask to be excused, and so I wet myself in the classroom instead.

My parents came from very different backgrounds, although ostensibly similar at the time of their marriage in the early 1950s. Then, sensible young women chose as their husbands men with prospects, and my father had just qualified as an architect. In the very act of marrying him, my mother could be said to have forsaken her own ambitions. She had talent as an artist, she went to art school, met my father and married young, thereafter devoting herself to her children and husband. Her parents were very conventional and upstanding. Her father was a stockbroker and her mother had pretensions to aristocracy, bestowed on her by the whispers that her father was an illegitimate child of the Earl of Lonsdale. My grandmother had always felt that she belonged in a noble milieu and that fate had dealt her a blow by placing her parent on the wrong side of the blanket. She was also a Catholic, and had renounced her faith in order to marry my Protestant grandfather.

My paternal great-great-grandfather, Henry Manning, was a tradesman who was made a Freeman of the City of London in 1856; in my waiting room there is a copy of an old scroll recording this fact. His son left the East End of London for North America to seek better prospects. He left behind a wife and three young boys hopeful that he would soon establish himself and be in a position to send for them. His ship foundered off the coast and he died of exposure after being recovered from the water.

Without a breadwinner, my grandfather learned to live by his wits. His father-in-law was a fine example of the prosperity this could bring. He had started out with minimal prospects, being a son of a farm labourer, and had gone on to become a professional gambler who made a fortune backing the right horses. Among his own string of twelve racehorses was one Scottish Grand National winner (Clydesdale, 1932). Due to the contacts he made through his father-in-law and his own interest in gambling and horse racing, my grandfather – a printer by trade – was able to produce a standardized rule-book for bookmakers in the late 1920s. Previously each bookmaker had printed his own set of rules by which bets could be made. My grandfather's initiative was to collate all the disparate rules and bind them into one book.

By the age of forty my grandfather had made enough money to enable him to retire. He did not work again, apart from dabbling in stocks, shares and property. In some respects he managed his wealth somewhat idiosyncratically. After his death my father discovered that he had been renting an iron for years, presumably because he had considered it a more efficient use of his money than buying one.

My father in a sense chose to break this adventurous mould. At the time of my birth, on 17 August 1955, he was working as an architect for a private practice in Cornwall. A short time later he was made redundant. He found a job with another firm, but when my mother was pregnant with my sister Rosalind, who is three years younger than me, he was made redundant again. At this point he decided it was his duty as a responsible father to have job security, so he accepted a position with what was then the East Anglian Regional Health Authority; in 1960 we moved to the other side of the country, to Shelford, a village about five miles outside Cambridge.

We did not have a television in our home. My father always said it was because we children would have spent all our time in front of it. In retrospect I think it was probably because he was afraid that he would have been the one to spend all his time looking at it! Because we did not have a television we had to find other ways of entertaining ourselves. In my case this resulted in me spending more time in my own head than other children might have done, dreaming things up. This world of the imagination was balanced by exposure to a very different environment.

When I was at primary school I became friends with a boy I shall always remember called Peter Townsend. He and I shared a desk. His father was a bricklayer, a countryman at heart who knew just about everything that could be known about wildlife. Peter and I would spend days wandering through the countryside looking at birds, their nests, butterflies and wild flowers. Thanks to those magical hours I can now identify almost every British bird and wild flower.

Looking back on it, my childhood seems strange and yet utterly normal. Life was more structured then, and if our lives were more rigidly structured than most, down to knowing in advance each week what we would be eating at every meal, it was only in degree. The perfectionist approach taken by my mother mirrored that of my father, who has always ordered his life, and finds it difficult to cope when his meticulous planning is upset. Probably most other families of our class lived in a similar way, because there was less choice, less diversity and more conformity.

By the early 1960s, when I was beginning to take notice of the world, the attitudes of the Fifties still held sway. People were expected to be models of restraint, resourcefulness and responsibility, and in the case of my parents, and probably millions of others like them, these expectations weighed heavily. The openness we now take for granted in the way people relate to each other was not acceptable then. In our family displays of affection were very rare, especially by my father.

I see my father now as a very fair, honest man, and the possessor of great spiritual qualities. I did not recognize any of this when I was younger, although had I looked I would have found evidence of them.

My father has always collected antiques. When we lived in Shelford he had a large collection of antique English coins. One Saturday we came back to the house to find that we had been burgled. Somebody had forced a window, got through it, and gone through every room in the house. It was discovered that my father's coin collection had been rifled and a number of valuable coins stolen.

The police came and took fingerprints and eventually arrested a fourteen-year-old boy, who had come from a children's home and been in the area selling flags for charity. Finding no one at home when he called at our house with his collection box, he had decided to break in. When the police asked the boy what he had done with the coins, he said that he had thrown some into the bushes, and some into the river. I remember my father being very upset by this. Being burgled was a hard enough fact for him to cope with, but to have a treasured possession taken and then treated with such disregard was doubly difficult.

The police asked my father if he wanted to press charges against the boy. My father is not a religious man, so his decision, that the police should severely caution him and then let him go, was not a learned response. He expressed the hope that if one of his children were ever to get into a similar situation, someone would make the same decision. That is, I think, on reflection, a spiritual response, and implicit in it is an understanding of how the right thought will beget the right deed.

I did not truly appreciate this side of my father until much later. In childhood I regarded him as a very logical man who rarely expressed emotion. His temper could be volcanic, and you could never be sure when it was going to explode or what might trigger it. I was aware of tension, friction and lack of emotional nurture in these early years, but not of their consequences.

This environment was my norm and I adapted to its shortfall, as children usually do. I was not able then to detect in it the seeds of problems that would arise later in my life and in the lives of my sister and brother. Nor did I suspect that it might be partly responsible for the series of peculiar happenings that began in our house in 1967. Only much later would I be able to identify them as the unruly offspring of sheer frustration and suppressed creativity that were bubbling away within each of us at an unconscious level.

✳   ✳   ✳

Our house in Shelford was not the kind traditionally associated with paranormal activity, being of recent, Fifties, construction and open plan in layout. We had lived there for seven years when the first outbreak occurred, one Saturday morning in February. My father went downstairs at seven o'clock to make up the fire of the all-night burning stove and discovered a Georgian silver tankard lying on the floor. This tankard was one of the many antique objects he had collected over the years, and was usually kept on a wooden shelf about four feet above the floor. We did not have a cat or dog so the culprit responsible for dislodging it could not have been an inquisitive or clumsy pet.

My father wondered if we had had burglars, but on checking the rest of the contents of the room he could find nothing missing. Using his architect's logic he examined the wooden shelf to see if warp might have caused the tankard to slide on to the

floor. This did not give him the practical answer he was looking
for. Puzzled, he questioned my younger sister and brother,
Rosalind and Andrew, and myself at breakfast. Each of us professed our ignorance of the happening. My father accepted our
word, and nothing more was said.

A few days later exactly the same thing happened. My father
came down to find the tankard on the floor. Again he checked
for evidence of burglars, and found none. Again we were questioned. This time we jokingly accused each other of being the
mischief maker. That night, unbeknown to us children, my
parents surreptitiously sprinkled talcum powder around the
tankard in the hope of tracing the manner of its going. Was the
tankard sliding off the shelf or jumping off it?

They found the answer the following morning: the tankard
was on the floor again, having negotiated the carefully sprinkled
ring of fine powder and left it undisturbed. There had been additional migrations too. A vase of jasmine in water had moved
some twenty feet across the room and was now sitting on the
table mat meant for the teapot; my mother had, as usual, laid
the table for breakfast the night before. A china dog had moved
from a shelf to a more prominent position above the fireplace, a
distance of about five feet.

I can remember our emotions being very mixed at this new
development. Childish amusement and delight mingled with fear.
Why were these strange tricks being played on us? What would
happen next? This was a time for questions, and yet perhaps
because we knew that our parents could not answer them, we
did not make it worse for them by persisting in asking the un-
answerable. My father did not know what to do or who to
approach but realized that we needed help of some kind. He
was quite certain that we were witnessing poltergeist activity.
(A poltergeist – literally, German for 'noisy spirit' – is a spirit that
makes its presence known by the displacement or removal of
solid objects, and frequently by loud noises.)

I am firmly of the belief that in some form or another we
receive the knowledge we need to make the decisions that

shape our lives. Many years previously, in his student days, my father had read a book called *Poltergeist Over England* by Harry Price. It was a very odd book to have read in those days, and even my father is not sure why he bought it. Interestingly, that book was never around in the house subsequently, so the knowledge it contained was not with us as a family, waiting to be picked up one wet Sunday afternoon and batted around as a topic of conversation.

My father's first attempt at bringing relief from what had quickly become almost daily occurrences was to approach the Departments of Child Psychology, Experimental Psychology and Clinical Psychology at Cambridge University. None of the people there believed him or were interested in what he had to tell them. Having drawn a blank there and not knowing who to turn to, he went one night to the police station in Cambridge to report that he had a poltergeist in the house. Quite what he thought the police were going do about it, I do not know, but it shows the level of his desperation.

There is a delightful synchronicity about this story, because on duty that night was a police sergeant whose all-consuming interest in life was psychical research. Far from belittling him with scepticism, the sergeant was fascinated by the story my father related to him. He knew immediately to whom my father should go for help. 'The man you need,' he said, 'is Professor George Owen.' My father had never heard of Professor Owen but gratefully took the sergeant's advice and contacted him.

Owen was a Professor of Genetics at Trinity College, Cambridge, and the world's leading expert on poltergeists. He had won, in 1963, The Treatise Award of the Parapsychology Foundation, and the following year was awarded the Duke University (in North Carolina) prize for distinguished work in parapsychology.

The professor lived conveniently close by, only five miles from our house, and within days of my father contacting him he came over to see us. He was impressively calm and collected, a welcome steadying influence after the spate of unnerving events we had been exposed to. A scientist through and through, he brought the same methodical, rational approach to parapsychology as he did to his conventional work in Cambridge.

It was an early lesson for me in the importance of acquiring a detached attitude, and for that I owe George Owen a great debt of gratitude. My father was greatly relieved to have found a man whose language and approach he understood and who did not regard him with suspicion. What my father described squared with the evidence Owen had gathered from his investigations of numerous poltergeist cases.

The house was, he thought, unlikely to be haunted, by virtue of its age. He assured us that what had happened was perfectly natural, although rare, and not the result of demonic intervention, possession or mental ill-health. Such activity, he told us, almost invariably occurred around children. The outbreak would last from between two and eight weeks, and once it had ceased it would not resume. He said that although poltergeists might be inconvenient – an understatement as it turned out later – they had great scientific interest. Reassured by his matter-of-fact approach, we set about making the best of what was becoming a very disconcerting way of life.

The person whose reaction I was most aware of during this period was my mother, perhaps because the similarity in our temperaments made me especially sensitive to her frame of mind and reactions to events. She became so frightened that she refused to stay in the house by herself during the day when we were at school and my father was at work. She would rather do anything than stay there alone, even if it was just wandering aimlessly around Cambridge window-shopping. At one point Professor Owen thought that she might be, in his words, 'the unconscious involuntary source of the force, as occasionally it is manifested by older persons, . . . because she was the one who seemed outwardly to be the most tense'.

My sister and brother were another matter. I was too involved in what was going on to notice their reactions. Although the events were affecting us as a unit, we did not share our fear, either with school friends or with each other. I told no one at school about what was going on at home. I did not want anyone to ostracize us or regard us as a peculiar family. Once we had recovered from the initial shock and fright, we tended to be British about it and treat it as a joke.

I did not realize the extent to which both Rosalind and Andrew were affected by what happened, and the potentially damaging trails it left in them, especially Andrew. He is still trying to dispel the immense fear he felt at the time, and now says that he felt 'raped' by the trauma of the events.

The line taken by Owen reinforced my father's dispassionate view of what we were faced with. His way of coping or making sense of it was to draw an architecturally to scale plan of the room in which the poltergeist activity was occurring. He would then log every movement of every object on these maps, recording what had moved and to where, the time the movement was discovered, and the estimated time the movement had occurred. The happenings always took place between 7 and 7.30 a.m., when we were just waking. My father was always the first to get up, so he would always be the one to discover the latest movements.

His plans show that the objects moved were invariably small, such as ashtrays, cutlery, baskets, plates. None of them was ever damaged or their contents spilt. The largest objects to move were a small coffee table and an armchair. The Georgian silver tankard was regularly moved, as was the vase of flowers. The tankard belonged to my father and he alone drank from it. Its movement could be read as some kind of defiant protest against him. Only recently have I come to see it as perhaps my way of breaking my father's very ordered, structured routine. The flowers were always placed on the breakfast table, in front of where my mother sat.

From the top of the stairs it was possible to hear knocks and other sounds, but we did not see the objects move, and it soon became clear that the objects would only move when no one was in the room. Owen undertook a small experiment of his own to satisfy himself that he was not being duped. He was already fairly certain of my father's integrity, but being a scientist he had to test every possible explanation.

Very early one morning he arrived unannounced on foot, having left his car some distance from the house, and took up a position outside from where he could see clearly into the living room. When nothing had happened by 7.15 a.m., he made his way into the house. He opened the door to the living room to find that, in the thirty seconds it had taken him to get there, several objects had been moved.

Owen and my father made several similar attempts to catch the poltergeist in the act, as it were. They would cordon off the room by fastening a series of cotton threads across the doorway, and then watch from positions outside the house. Always they would see nothing and then go inside to find the threads undisturbed and objects in different positions.

On 6 March, about a fortnight after the first happening, George Owen suggested to my parents that we children be sent individually to stay with friends. In this way he hoped to identify which of us might be the involuntary source of the activity. This experiment was inconclusive, in that no poltergeist activity occurred either in the house or where we were staying while we were away, although my parents reported that the erratic taps and creaks which had started up soon after the first happening had still been audible at all hours of the day.

It was not mentioned to me at the time, but George Owen thought I was the most likely member of the family around whom the poltergeist activity centred, largely on account of my age. (I was eleven years six months old, Rosalind was eight years seven months and Andrew was seven years old.) I was shortly to sit the Common Entrance Examination, and the result of this would decide which school I went to after I left my preparatory school.

Owen believed that my anxiety at having to clear this first major hurdle in my academic career might be a contributory factor in generating the energy responsible for the outbreak. He was in no doubt, as he wrote later to my father, after the activity had died down, that: 'The force, whatever it may be, resides principally in Matthew'.

Our return home was greeted with a rush of activity. On the first morning nine objects moved, among them an upholstered chair, which moved about six feet, a dining chair, which was turned upside down, and a candlestick, which was placed in the middle of a vase of flowers. The following morning marked the peak of activity during this outbreak. Eleven objects were moved during a period of fifteen minutes. The last of these movements was the most unnerving. My sister Rosalind was in the living room, sketching. She reached for her rubber to correct a mistake, but could not find it. At this point I entered the room and saw the rubber rising up from behind the sofa on which she was sitting. Almost in the same instant Rosalind became aware of it too. We watched, transfixed, as the rubber moved slowly towards her and landed beside her on the sofa. Without exchanging a word, we bolted from the room.

After this exhibition of the poltergeist's helpfulness, objects moved shorter distances and gradually the movements stopped altogether. George Owen had assured us that the activity would cease, never to return, and after three months it seemed that was the case. We went on holiday at Easter, came back three weeks later and found that life had returned to normal. There were no more inexplicable creaks, groans and pings, and objects stayed put. Gradually, too, we lost the habit of constantly looking over our shoulders.

✳   ✳   ✳

In the autumn of 1968 we moved to the eighteenth-century Queen's House at Linton, some eight miles away from our previous home. The move coincided with another major upheaval, my going away from home for the first time, to Oakham School in Rutland. It took some time for me to get used to the spartan, regimented environment at the school. I did not like the place at all in the beginning, not least because a system of fagging (in which first-year boys act as unpaid servants to senior boys) was still in operation; it had been abolished by the time I reached an age where I could make use of it.

The school had a very military feel to it, due to the fact that most of the staff were retired army officers. In my first term I was perceived to be withdrawn and nervous, and lacking in self-confidence. Survival, I decided, depended on keeping my head down and attracting as little attention to myself as possible. By the following year, I was still 'very shy', according to my house-master, but 'perfectly happy'. Little did he know how much I hated the lack of privacy, the bare floors and always feeling cold.

One advantage I had over other boys in that first year was that I had gone to Oakham with a ready-made friend, Andrew Dickson, who had been at prep school with me. He became my closest friend in my teenage years, and was something of a foil for me. Whereas I was shy and retiring, he was bold and outgoing. Both of us wanted to travel, but he made it possible.

After our first year at Oakham we started exploring Britain together, hitchhiking with sleeping bags and a tent. I would not have had the confidence to do it by myself, but with Andrew it was easy. He was much more worldly wise and mature than I was. Nothing daunted him. Our lives have gone in parallel in some senses. He qualified as a doctor and has spent his life trav-elling, as indeed have I.

In my school work it quickly became apparent where my strengths and weaknesses lay: my enthusiasm for English and History matched my ability in both subjects. This contrasted markedly with my dislike of the subjects the school prized most highly – Maths and the sciences – and the correspondingly poor results I achieved in them. Boys of my age were expected to be methodical and to enjoy mastering formulas and constructs, but my mind simply did not work like that – it still doesn't. I came across as diffident, lacking in application and a bit of a dreamer. I held my own, but I did not fit in. I felt like a peculiarity, an outsider. This became obvious to everyone else at school in the spring term of 1971.

I had taken two English O Levels in the summer term of 1970, which left six further O Levels to be taken the following year. This was my objective when I returned home for the long summer break in July. A few days after my return my parents bought a very large oak wardrobe for my bedroom, which was placed on the ground floor of the house. At some point in its life the wardrobe had been cut in half, presumably to make it easier to shift.

I regarded this new acquisition with mixed feelings. I liked it and yet felt there was something wrong with it. I put my clothes in it and closed it, fastening the left-hand door top and bottom by means of its two bolts, and securing the right-hand door to the left by turning a key-operated lock. A few minutes later I came back to the room to fetch something and found both doors open.

I looked for a simple explanation. Perhaps the halves of the wardrobe were not screwed tightly together, and they were slipping their respective bolts and lock, but I could not find any evidence for this. I rebolted and locked the doors and left the room for a second time. When I came back a third time, again the doors were wide open. This went on for several days. The doors would never open spontaneously while I was in the room, only when I was absent. My parents seemed uninterested when I told them what was happening.

I returned to school in September no nearer to discovering why the wardrobe doors seemed to have a life of their own. The strange activity continued the next time I went home. The wardrobe doors were closed when I first entered the room and when I left it after unpacking. When I went back subsequently they were open. I closed them and sat down to listen to a record. After about fifteen minutes a boot shot across the room from the direction of the wardrobe, which was behind me, and hit the window about ten feet in front of me. I looked around and there were the doors, wide open. I said nothing about this, and the rest of the weekend passed without a recurrence.

On my next visit home, at half-term, the cushions in my bedroom floated from one side to the other and coat hangers started to move too. Later they would nudge me gently from behind. I found these movements more irritating than frightening, because I seemed to be the only one in the house who was being subjected to them. My parents remained resolutely uninterested on the few occasions I did venture to mention what was occurring in my room.

On Christmas morning I heard scratching which seemed to be coming from behind the panelling on the other side of the room. This faded away to be replaced by a noise just outside the window that sounded like someone walking up and down on gravel. I got up and looked out of the window, expecting to see footprints in the snow, but there were none; there was no gravel there either. No sooner had I got back into bed than the scratching noise started again. I went to fetch my mother so she could hear with her own ears that something peculiar was going on. All was quiet when we entered the room together and she refused to believe my story, insisting that George Owen had said these things did not come back.

School was the one place where I seemed safe from the poltergeist activity. This changed quietly, almost imperceptibly. First my pen went missing from the desk in my study, and then turned up in the study next door. The three boys who shared that study denied taking it, so I thought I must have left it behind without realizing, although I could not remember visiting their room recently. A short time later the pen went missing again, and this time was found in a different study further away. Other objects of mine also started to roam. I could not prove beyond a shadow of a doubt that these items had not been removed by another person.

The first conclusive evidence of paranormal activity occurred one night when I was in the study listening to music with the two other boys I shared with. I got up to change the record and as I pushed the automatic switch to operate the arm, the record on the turntable began to rise slowly up the centre shaft, revolving in an anti-clockwise direction as it ascended. The record jammed when it reached the top of the shaft and I had great difficulty in dislodging it. None of us could begin to explain what had happened before our eyes.

A few days after I came home for the Easter holidays in April 1971 my parents began to notice that objects were moving again, but said nothing. I had got used to keeping quiet about what was happening around me so there we were, individually aware while pretending not to be. The pretence stopped on the evening of Easter Sunday. My parents were entertaining friends who arrived at the house while I was out. I got home shortly before they were about to leave, around ten o'clock, and went straight to bed.

As my parents were showing their guests out, they were embarrassed by the sight of a large pewter plate turned upside down on the dining-room table. Their guests probably did not notice this oddity as they passed through, but my parents have always been very precise about the siting and placing of orna-ments. It did not escape their attention either, when they went back into the lounge where they had been entertaining, that the sofa had moved and was now on the other side of the room. They knew Rosalind and Andrew had been in bed for several hours and that I was in my room, so none of us could have been responsible for shifting it.

While my parents were puzzling over these events, I was in bed taking part in what I can only describe as a scene worthy of a horror film. I was lying there feeling restless when suddenly I heard a creaking noise coming from the wardrobe on the other side of the room. I switched on the light and to my amazement saw the wardrobe inching out from the wall towards me. It advanced about eighteen inches before I panicked and switched off the light. I did not want to see this; it could carry on without me as a spectator. Then my bed started to vibrate and the feet rose into the air. I just lay there terrified, not knowing what to do. The head end started to move up as well until I was completely airborne about six inches off the ground. Finally, the bed shot round and ended up at an angle to the wall.

Enough was enough. I did not want to sleep in this room any longer. I got out of bed and went to find my parents. They had

their own secrets to impart, and told me about the recent movements they had noticed. The three of us then went to my bedroom.
The force that had been at work while I was in bed had also been
productive during the few minutes I was away from the room: a
heavy armchair had been moved and was now blocking the
doorway, physically preventing us from entering the room.

I spent the rest of the night in a sleeping bag on the floor of
my parents' bedroom, worrying about what might happen next.
Nothing untoward did happen during the long hours before
morning, so we had no intimation of the explosion of activity
that must have occurred at some point that night, in the kitchen,
the sitting room and the dining room. At first sight it looked as
though these parts of the house had played host to the sort of
exaggerated ruck you get in an old-fashioned Western – tables
and chairs had been upturned or were piled on top of each other,
and objects were strewn all over the floors. The only element
missing was damage. Nothing was broken. The intent was obviously not to injure either our possessions or our feelings.

We started to impose some order on this seemingly mischie-
vous, carefully contrived chaos, but no sooner did we succeed in
putting one room to rights then, in a matter of minutes and
behind our backs, it was returned to its chaotic state. We were
condemned to spending the whole of Easter Monday playing
this frustrating game.

This was our induction to a kind of will-o'-the-wisp poltergeist
activity we had not experienced before. Over the next few days
beds were stripped completely or overturned. One morning my
brother and sister were met at the kitchen door by a trolley gliding
towards them about an inch off the floor. We would find objects
perched precariously in unlikely places: a broom balanced hori-
zontally across the handrail of our staircase; three metal-framed
tables with stone tops placed delicately one on top of the other.

We would discover pools of water, a phenomenon mostly
limited to one area of stone floor in the hall. Then the poltergeist
began to use other types of liquid from containers in the house:
ink, acid and paint stripper were all at one time poured on to the

floor. On one occasion we suspected that it had employed sodium hydroxide crystals – from a jar kept in the cellar – in a liquid poured over the linoleum covering the floor in a room upstairs. When this mischief was discovered the linoleum was in the process of dissolving and we burned our hands as we tried to mop up the substance with cloths.

My father decided to seek out George Owen again for advice, but he was by this time the Director of The New Horizons Research Foundation in Toronto, and thousands of miles away from our predicament. It seemed there was nothing we could do but watch as this vigorous force tried to take over our lives. After about two weeks it became clear that the activity was basically divisible into three categories: the first was purely disruptive and annoying; the second was concerned with symmetry and balance, and the third was boisterous, noisy movement, designed it seemed, to attract attention.

The third type was the most interesting, because we were allowed to witness it as it happened. Objects would first vibrate and then shake violently before rising into the air and moving away. Once airborne the objects would pick up speed, especially as they approached the stairs. When they reached the bottom of these they would be hurled up to the top with terrific force. Sometimes objects would hit walls and land noisily on the floor. Hammers, mallets, coat hangers, blocks of wood, gallon cans of paint stripper and carpentry tools all at some time or another crashed during these airborne manoeuvres. Sometimes, though, objects would be moved with great care and precision, negotiating the two right-angles on the staircase leading up to the first floor and lobbing themselves over the handrail at the top.

The most startling example of this kind of movement occurred one afternoon, when it was discovered that the table in my sister's room was no longer there. This table had a drawer in it and was about twenty-nine inches high by thirty-six inches long by eighteen inches wide. She used it as a study desk and kept on it books, papers, a mug of pencils and assorted ornaments. Our first search for it drew a blank. We searched again, this time taking in the cellar. To our astonishment there was the table. None of the objects on it was out of place, although somehow it must have been negotiated down three flights of stairs, and through five doorways, some less than thirty inches wide, and ten complete right-angled changes of direction, in order to reach the cellar.

During the first few days of the outbreak childlike scribbles, circles and doodles had appeared on walls throughout the house, usually executed with a lead pencil. A little later we saw on the walls the words, 'Matthew Beware', and what appeared to be the astrological sign for Leo (my birth sign). I tried not to think too hard about what this warning might mean. What we were being subjected to was worrying enough without it becoming somehow personalized. When a short time later the same warning appeared again, my mother suggested that I might put a piece of paper and a pencil on the dining-room table and invite the poltergeist to use them. I thought her idea a good one and did as she suggested.

We closed the curtains to give the poltergeist the privacy it seemed to require, and went upstairs, locking the door to the room as we withdrew; no one else was in the house. We returned to the room ten minutes later. On the sheet was a series of indecipherable scribblings. I took another sheet of paper and wrote across the top the alphabet and the numbers 0 to 9. We left the sheet on the table and withdrew again. When we came back we found more small scribblings, a Leo sign and in the centre the words 'Matthew Beware'.

This exercise seemed to prove beyond doubt that I was the source of the energy feeding the poltergeist. At about this time we became aware of another important aspect of the phenome-non. One day my mother asked me to move a small wicker basket from the kitchen table to the dining-room table. We were both upstairs when she asked me to do this. We went down-stairs together to find that the poltergeist had performed the task for me: the wicker basket was now sitting in the middle of the dining-room table.

On the day before I was due back at school for the start of the summer term my parents asked me if I could try to get back some of the objects that seemed to have gone missing during the poltergeist activity. None of these objects was valuable so much as useful, like teaspoons or crockery. We were all in the sitting room at the time, and I suggested that we stay where we were while I tried to get the articles returned to the table in the dining room. Half an hour later we went into the dining room and were amazed to find an array of objects, many of which my parents had not even noticed as being missing. Table mats, books, ornaments, in addition to the humble spoons and crockery initially requested, had been placed neatly on the table.

My father thought it only fair to warn my headmaster, John Buchanan, of the possibility of the poltergeist activity we had experienced during the holiday also occurring at Oakham. Mr Buchanan had never encountered anything of the nature described to him by my father. He was slightly dismissive and believed that, 'in the hurly burly of school life', nothing much would happen in a large dormitory shared with twenty-five other boys. His ignorance at this point was perhaps a blessing. My father had visions of him turfing me out and no other comparable school wanting to find a place for me.

It was decided that I should be given a bunk bed to myself and that this should be placed away from the other beds, in a corner of the large, square dormitory, by a window. The first night passed uneventfully. Shortly after lights out on the second night I felt the bed move towards the centre of the room. I got out and pushed it back the eighteen or so inches it had advanced. Within a couple of minutes it was on the move again, and this time several other boys saw what was going on. I decided not to push it back. An empty bunk then began to move sideways towards a block of beds. It moved about six feet and stopped. My bed decided to follow it, eventually stopping after about four feet. At this point one of the astonished observers in the other beds switched on the lights. We returned the beds to their original positions and turned out the lights. When my bed moved out from the wall again, I left it where it was.

The same movements occurred on the following night, and on the night after that. The dormitory was soon buzzing with chatter as we boys tried to work out how this could be happening. The bunks had heavy metal frames with rubber-bottomed feet and were difficult to move empty, let alone when they had someone lying in them. After this third episode a friend of mine went to the matron and told her what had occurred. When the headmaster was told, he decided not to do anything because the disturbance was on a small scale and confined to one dormitory.

The poltergeist displays increased over the following days. As well as bunks moving when the lights were out, objects were now being hurled across the room. When we turned on the lights we found pieces of broken glass, screws and nails littering the floor. We swept the floor and left the debris in the corner. As we settled down to sleep again the debris was redistributed all around the room. That same night the contents of my study were turned upside down.

The same mayhem occurred during the following night. Various items, such as pebbles, broken glass, cutlery and pieces of wood, were flung around the dormitory, and especially against the walls and windows. The dormitory had no curtains, and by this time all the boys in the room were on the lookout for anyone who might be responsible for the havoc being wrought on them every night. The morning after it was discovered that the studies of other boys had been disturbed, with bookcases emptied and pieces of furniture upturned. There were also pools of water on large areas of the floors.

After this burst of activity Mr. Buchanan was as desperate as I was to stop what was going on. He decided to take the matron's advice and consult someone experienced in these matters. The matron had more than a passing interest in the paranormal and, as well as having contacts with mediums and psychics, was probably the least fazed by what was going on. An appointment was made for me to see the man recommended by her in a week's time. This was too long a wait for the headmaster. Some attempt at intervention had to be made immediately, he felt. He asked the school chaplain if he could be of assistance, but the chaplain freely admitted during our short chat that it was beyond him to offer a solution to the present problem. He had heard of such happenings, but could offer no help and did not even hazard an opinion as to what such paranormal happenings might signify.

The days between Mr Buchanan making the appointment and my keeping it brought a variety of poltergeist activity in the dormitory. One night nothing but glass would be hurled around the room, the next it would be only nails. Other items included skewers, stones, pieces of broken concrete and spoons. Particularly terrifying was the night when bone-handled knives were thrown against walls and beds. Several times boys were struck by them, although very gently and without causing them harm. In the morning we collected the knives from where they lay on the floor. There were fourteen of them, all bearing a royal crest and the initials GR. They did not belong to the school and we were unable to establish their origin.

A couple of days after this we were treated to an aerial display by twenty metal coat hangers. When we found them in the morning they appeared as small balls of squashed heavy-gauge wire.

Mr Buchanan did not see any of this activity for himself but in a BBC documentary in 1985 he reported that he had 'received numerous first-hand stories from the boys and from the house tutor and the matron.' Peter Weight, the house tutor in question, recalled what he had witnessed:

I remember one boy being terrified because a glow of light appeared on a wall which seemed to be warm to the touch. Objects began to fly through the air in the dormitories and appear on the floor: knives, forks, bits of broken china, this kind of thing. On one occasion a whole pile of dinner plates from the dining hall seemed to appear from nowhere and crashed to the floor.

We did check out one of the things which was happening. Every day the boys had to make their beds in the
dormitory. These were normally inspected by the prefects
as soon as they had been made. After doing this the
prefects went off to school, at about five to nine. At about
five past nine it was the custom of the matron to go
round the dormitories and check the beds for herself.

For a number of weeks most of the beds in the dormitories were in disarray. They were all topsy-turvy,
mattresses half off the beds, the sheets all over the place.
Obviously we thought someone must be coming back
and doing this as a kind of prank, but it seemed to happen
over and over again. As far as we could judge, nobody was
about the House at the time.

On one occasion – and this did frighten me – I was away
for a half-term and came back. My room was at the end of
a corridor. I had a large, heavy suitcase which I put on top
of a large chest of drawers, and left various other bits and
pieces around. Then I went off to have supper. When I
returned it looked to me as though a giant hand had
simply picked up everything in the room and dropped it
back down again. Now, if someone had been in the room
and disarrayed it, they might have thrown the things
around, but from the position of the suitcase, the way the
mattress was, and so on, it really looked more like either
a wind or something had picked them up and dropped
them down. That particular night I did not sleep very well.

The incident with the glow of light referred to by Mr. Weight
occurred in the early hours of the Saturday on which I was to be
taken to the man on whom the headmaster was pinning his
hopes. A prefect – a close friend of mine at the time – in a dormitory in another part of Deanscroft House woke up at 4.30 a.m.
feeling icy cold. On the wall opposite him he saw a disc of
luminous light about eighteen inches in diameter. At first he
thought it was being projected into the room from the corridor

outside. The chill in the air intensified, and as it did so the area
of light increased, gradually extending from the skirting board
to the ceiling and to about six feet in width across the wall. Half
an hour later the matron found the boy on his knees in the
corridor, praying. The light had almost disappeared when she
returned to the dormitory with him.

That same day, 8 May 1971, my house tutor took me to a mental
hospital in nearby Leicester to keep the appointment made by the
headmaster. We were shown into a small room where a man was
sitting with a dark-haired woman. I had taken along a basket full
of apports to show him, but he barely glanced at them and he did
not seem interested in what I wanted to say about what was happening. He had the answer, which I was to copy down from the
small book he handed me. I should perform this banishing ritual
every time something paranormal occurred, he said.

> Face east. Touch forehead and say ATEH (thou art). Touch
> breast and say MALKUTH (The Kingdom). Touch right
> shoulder and say VE-GEBURAH (and the Power). Touch
> left shoulder and say VE-GEDULAH (and the Glory). Clasp
> hands before you and say LE-OLAM (forever). Point up
> and say AMEN. Make in the air toward the East the ban-
> ishing Pentagram, vibrate the deity name – YOD HE VAU
> HE. Imagine your voice carries forward to the East of the
> Universe. Hold out finger before you, go to South, make
> the Pentagram and vibrate similarly the deity name
> ADONAI. Go to West, make Pentagram and vibrate
> EHEIEH. Go to North, make the Pentagram and vibrate
> AGLA. Return to East and complete your circle by
> bringing the finger point to centre of the first Pentagram.
> Stand with arms outstretched in the form of a cross and
> say – Before me Raphael (Air), Behind me Gabriel (Water),
> at my right hand Michael (Fire), at my left hand Auriel
> (Earth). Before me flames the Pentagram, behind me
> shines the siX-rayed star. Make again the Quabalistic Cross
> as directed above saying ATEH, etc.

My sense of the ridiculous almost got the better of me. Given that every day brought a rash of paranormal happenings, I could envisage spending all my time uttering his mumbo-jumbo. This at a time when I was trying to study for the six O Levels I was expected to sit in a few weeks. I kept my reservations to myself and dutifully took down the ritual.

The man and the woman represented my first brush with occult practitioners. During the subsequent hour and a half we spent with them they demonstrated impressive clairvoyant skills in giving both of us accurate character and life readings. The man told us about his experiences with astral projection, and explained how it was done.

I neither liked nor trusted this man. The whiff of the sorcerer clung to him, and this insulted my youthful pride. He represented an aspect of psychism that repelled me, and still does – the gathering and practice of secret knowledge for its own sake. This narrow, individualistic approach has, I believe, damaged the credibility of the paranormal, by shrouding the subject in unnecessary mysticism, closing it off from view by the many and keeping it the preserve of a cranky few.

We left the meeting unsure whether we had been on a fool's errand. The man had been most peculiar, we both agreed. Anyway, I decided not to let my personal opinion of him prejudice me against his advice. That evening I went up to the dormitory and performed the ritual, taking special care to draw the pentagrams the right way round. If I drew them the wrong way, even inadvertently, I risked invoking a force.

Within two hours it looked as though I might have done just that, because havoc was ensuing. I repeated the ritual a second time, and a third. It was obvious that peace would only be restored if I left the dormitory. I determined not to sleep there and decided that the wisest course of action would be to spend the night in Matron's sitting room. Whatever happened, she could be relied upon not to panic.

Word quickly got around and by bedtime the matron had a group of anxious boys around her in the downstairs washroom.

As she tried to calm their fears and reassure them, a plug hurtled across from an empty corner of the room and landed at her feet. Several pieces of broken glass then tumbled from the ceiling. The whole group was shaken, although in Matron's case the cause was excitement rather than terror.

I had a strong feeling more was to come. A few other boys joined Matron and myself in her sitting room. We chatted until about 11.30, when they left to go to bed; Matron and myself were left to continue the vigil.

Shortly after the boys had left, wood chippings, small pebbles and pieces of glass appeared in our laps and fell into our cups of coffee. Knocking noises emanated from the walls, ceiling and floor, and pinging sounds came from the windows, pictures and even cups. Eventually the materializations stopped and all the sounds, except for a rapping on the walls, died down.

Matron went off to do her final round of all the dormitories. Everywhere was quiet and undisturbed. She returned to the sitting room where I was waiting and sat down. The rapping noises on the walls were still audible and had been throughout her absence. Then, simultaneously, we felt a curious freezing sensation around our feet and lower legs, which gradually crept up our bodies. This became so uncomfortable that we were forced to shift our positions. Once we moved the sensation disappeared.

We took this as a sign that something was about to happen, and went next door to the small dormitory housing eight of the younger boys and two older prefects. As we entered the room we both experienced the same chill that had crept over us earlier and saw a small patch of light on the wall facing us. There was no outside source that could be causing this.

I went up to the patch and placed my hand in front of it to see if I could make a shadow. None appeared. I touched the patch. It felt warm and contrasted sharply with the areas outside it, which were as cool as one would expect uncovered plaster to be. The boy above whose head the circle had formed woke up, aware of the chill around him. He saw the bright light and watched with us as the patch expanded. I saw what looked like a crown of thorns form around its edge. Interestingly, the matron saw a different image – a cross over the light.

I performed the banishing ritual, this time focusing my thoughts on removing the light from the wall. After twenty minutes the patch of light had shrunk to the size of a saucer and the images around it were no longer visible. As the paranormal light dimmed the temperature in the room returned to normal. When the electric light was switched on the paranormal light faded completely.

Later that morning I was told of Mr Buchanan's decision to ask my parents to come that very afternoon and discuss my future at the school. After four weeks of 'something very peculiar going on', having to deal with a chorus of enquiries from worried parents, and having little evidence that the banishing ritual was the answer, he was at his wits' end. The last thing he wanted was for parents to start complaining and the whole business being brought to the attention of the press.

I sympathized. I seemed to be the cause of the problem, and the simplest solution would be to remove me. Almost without exception the boys in my house did not blame me for what was happening, and they defended me against the scepticism shown by boys from other houses. They were in the main a stoical, supportive bunch, and their attitude made the situation easier for me than it might have been. In the words of one of the boys in my dormitory, when questioned by David Frost on his show in 1974, it was 'something we got used to after a while. It was commonplace.'

I can recall being frightened on only two occasions: when the wardrobe moved and when the circle of light appeared on the wall. The situation was helped by the benign nature of the poltergeist. There was never a sense of menace. We did not worry about the fact that what was happening defied rational explanation. The grown-ups worried on our behalf.

My housemaster, Roger Blackmore, was 'primarily concerned to prevent boys in the house becoming over-conscious of what might be going on, exaggerating it. And, indeed, I felt for

Matthew himself. I hoped very much that he wouldn't be suffering as a result of what people were saying about him or his own misgivings about what was happening.'

When I told Matron of my imminent removal she thought it most unjust and was intent on trying to dissuade the headmaster. While we were discussing this new development, there was a knock on the door. A prefect who had been checking the dormitories came in and handed her two things that he had found near my bed. The first was a length of wire twisted into a ring the size of a saucer. The second was a grey, soft-bound booklet which had on its cover an illustration of a crucifix with a crown of thorns – an amalgamation of the images matron and I had seen on the wall during the night. The booklet was a copy of 'The Saint John and Saint Matthew Passion'.

By mid-morning John Buchanan had undergone a change of heart. I could stay at the school, he told my father. The worst, he thought, was now behind us.

My parents were particularly concerned about the psychological effect the poltergeist activity might be having on me and the other pupils. At my father's request, George Owen wrote to the headmaster, urging him to bring the subject into the open and address the school. This approach would, in his opinion, 'be useful in lowering the temperature'. He suggested a template for such an address:

These events, though rare, do occur more often than is supposed. They are not due to tricks, or people 'seeing things'. They are due to unusual physical forces which people sometimes develop. These forces are the subject of active study by scientists in England, U.S.A., Canada and Europe. The best authorities believe them to be natural though rare. They are not supernatural. This particular case is one of a kind that happens somewhere in the world every few months. . . . Many people have rare talents, e.g. hearing other people's thoughts. Others have the ability to move objects by the unknown force. When talents start up like this it is scientifically extremely important and interesting.

It seems to me now that Buchanan's decision to, in his own words, 'play it at as low a key as possible' contributed to the 'build-up of consternation and . . . dismay'. As in other areas of life, concealment allows misconceptions to flourish. The strange man at the psychiatric hospital in Leicester and the fairly square and sceptical Mr Buchanan seemed to represent the opposite poles of opinion, between which the subject of the paranormal was uncomfortably stretched.

On the same afternoon that my parents came to the school, Matron received a call from the man in Leicester. He told her that he had invoked the light on the wall and that he had travelled astrally to the room, where he had seen both of us. The banishing ritual, he said, was my key to controlling the energy currently presenting as poltergeist activity.

In the circumstances there was little I could do but continue to carry out the ritual. Although the activity seemed to be lessening, enough strange incidents were being reported to panic the headmaster into again holding the threat of removal over my head.

I remember spending a miserable night, thinking about my family and wanting to tell my parents that it was not my fault I was being asked to leave again. I thought, 'If the poltergeist would only happen around Rosalind as well, they wouldn't be able to blame just me.' Later Rosalind told me that on that fretful night she had woken in the early hours to find her pillow in a corner on the opposite side of the room and her alarm clock under her bed.

Matron persuaded Buchanan against carrying out his threat, and once more I was reprieved. However, I knew intuitively that I should take steps to curb this force and should not wait passively for the next odd occurrence. In a recent letter to my father, George Owen had theorized on what might happen in the immediate future so far as the poltergeist was concerned. He had written:

> **With Matthew the following different possibilities can happen:**
>
> 1. The powers, whether voluntary or involuntary, may disappear suddenly.
>
> 2. He may retain them and achieve a high degree of control.
>
> 3. Most of the phenomena may vanish, but he may be left with one or two capacities.

I wondered which of George Owen's categories I fitted. My father, meanwhile, voiced his concern over what sort of life I could expect, especially within the framework of scenario two. Marital strife was a foregone conclusion because I could never be deceived. Every little white lie would be exposed in a flash of recognition – imagine the trouble, he would say, if my wife told me she had spent ten shillings and sixpence on a hat and I knew intuitively it had been twice as much.

I would let him ramble on, more amused than bothered by this prospect. Deep down, I wanted to be included in that second category he feared so much. I wanted to find out more, to go further, to decide my own future. I was curious to discover how many powers I did possess; indeed, to discover how many there were. Could I, for example, emulate the man in Leicester, and project myself astrally?

I decided to put myself to the test and attempt to 'travel' home. I lay down on my bed and thought about our house. I did not obviously 'travel' there so much as daydream about it. My impressions included: entering the open back door, seeing my mother standing at the sink by the washing machine; her looking in my direction, then turning back to her chores; following her into the dining room, and seeing her turn around to look intently at the spot where I was standing; following her around the house as she wandered from room to room, stopping occasionally to gaze thoughtfully in my direction. At the end of this experiment I was not sure what I had succeeded in doing, apart from giving myself a headache that lasted several days.

On my next weekend home, I told my mother about my 'journey'. She said that she had felt my presence in the house on that Monday morning, and that she had half-expected to see me, although she knew this was highly improbable because I was at school. Her experience encouraged me to take the experiment one stage further. This time I would try to project myself back in time. I thought I would be more likely to succeed if I carried out the experiment in our house, which had been built in stages between 1550 and 1730.

I worked out in advance the questions I would ask if I succeeded in my aim. The man in Leicester had told me that the first question to ask when communicating with spirits was, 'Do you come in peace?' I had no idea whether this would be any more effective than his banishing ritual, but it seemed sensible to err on the side of caution. I lay down and concentrated as before. Unlike on that first occasion, however, this time I seemed to enter naturally into a trance-like state. After a while a soft voice sounded somewhere near my head.

'Do you come in peace?'
'Yes.'
'What is your name?'
'Henrietta. Henrietta Webb.'
'When were you born?'
'In the year of Our dear Lord, sixteen hundred and nineteen.'
'Whom did you marry?'
'James Webb.'
'What was his trade?'
'He traded woollen drapery.'
'When did you first occupy this building?'
'In the year sixteen hundred and forty-six.'
'What were the names of your children?'

'Henrietta, James, Ellen, and Anne and Charles.'

'When did you die?'

There was a long pause before she replied, 'I passed away in the year of Our Lord sixteen hundred and seventy-three. I beg of you to pray for my spirit.'

'And from what did you die?'

'A poor fever.'

I asked her what kind of fever, but she did not reply.

'Where did your husband trade?'

'He traded from Butchers Row and Hog Lane.'

'What do you think of this house since you left it?'

She did not seem to grasp this question and made some comment about the noise. Then I lost contact with her.

Sometime later, I could hear another voice:

'Here am I. Here is Thomas.'

'Thomas who?'

'Yea, Thomas Salmon.'

'When were you born?'

'I was born of Thomas and Mary in the year fifteen hundred and sixty-eight.'

'To whom were you married?'

'My dear Rachel.'

His voice then disappeared, to be replaced almost immediately by that of another man who introduced himself as Richard Webb, a gentleman farmer, who did not know when he was born. He had married a Mistress Anne Thyson and had come into possession of the house in 1688.

Shortly after he broke off contact, I seemed to come back to the present. I had begun the experiment at 10.45 p.m. The time was now past two in the morning. I felt tired but was eager to see if I could make further contacts. I went back into a trance and soon heard:

'Anne. Anne. Here is Anne Willis.'

'When were you born?'

'Seventeen hundred and two.'

'Whom did you marry?'

'Robert was my husband. Robert Webbe.'

'What was Robert's trade?'

'A trader in grain was Robert.'

'When did you first occupy the house? Did Robert have the front of the house built?'

'Yes. Robert had this house builded in October in seventeen hundred and thirty. His fine house.'

After this statement her voice faded. I became aware that it was growing lighter in the room. Then I found myself standing in our hallway, in what appeared to be broad daylight. How flat and clean the stone floor looked, I thought, not at all worn as I knew it to be. I was puzzled by a heavy door opening onto a courtyard, and realized that I must be viewing the house as it had been in the early part of the eighteenth century. A child in a full-length dress was learning to walk with the aid of a cane frame on wheels. On the stairs a man was kneeling in a corner, hammering silently. He had gingery hair and wore a long leather apron.

As I moved from the hallway into the dining room, I was struck by the vivid blue of the plastered wall above the panelling on the staircase. In the dining room the fireplace that I was familiar with as bare brick was plastered and significantly lower. All the windows were leaded and not wooden framed. The room itself appeared to have one window fewer. A dog sprawled across the hearth paid me no more attention than had the little girl and the man. The next thing I knew I was wide awake on my bed. I wrote down my impressions immediately to minimize the risk of distortions to the experience, then went to bed.

We had four days of complete peace after my return to school the following evening. The poltergeist activity resumed after this respite but was less violent than before. This state of affairs was preferable to what we had grown used to but it was not satisfactory to me. I wanted the phenomena to stop completely.

I continued with the banishing ritual, although it seemed to be having no effect, and thought about what I should try next. The answer presented itself while I was writing an essay. The topic of this essay escapes me now, but it was obviously not one I relished because ideas came very slowly. I had to force them out of my head and on to the paper. As I was sitting, pen poised, musing over what to put, suddenly my hand was pushed down on to the paper and I started to scrawl words I did not understand in illegible handwriting. This shook me and I immediately tore up the piece of paper.

When I had recovered my composure, I assessed what had happened. Something had obviously been using me as a means of communication. On 6 June I asked a few of my school friends to witness an experiment I would be conducting that evening in my study. We sat with the lights out. I held a pen above a sheet of paper and concentrated on offering myself as a channel for automatic writing. Ten minutes passed and nothing happened. I tried again, this time adjusting the position of my hand so the pen was resting on the paper rather than hovering above it. Soon I felt the pen being guided across the paper.

On this occasion as on all subsequent occasions when I was engaged in automatic writing, I was not consciously aware of what was being written. I had to read it through afterwards to find out. The short sentence in a spidery hand read:

'I need help now. You cannot get me. Help. Please.'
Then I got: 'Danger. Stop. If you do not you will . . . 5 am not knife.'

Confused, I wrote on the paper: 'Who is this?'

'Joseph West 1783. Get the dog. I need you to help soon. Fire. Fire. Fire 11 June. I too high so die when I need your help soon. Danger of fire when coot dog. Get me soon I beg you.'

The writing became illegible and I asked the entity to explain further. The answer came back:

'See your bed too late when into the fire. Do not get the dog on the 19th June. Glass to be dropped into fire. Get fields on 19th June past second you and get it with you two.'

The message seemed to be breaking up, as sometimes happens on mobile phones when you receive only a few words out of whole sentences. Nonetheless, I seemed to have succeeded in producing writing that had possibly originated outside myself. My six witnesses went to bed shortly afterwards. Three of them found their beds wet inside.

No poltergeist activity occurred for three days after this episode. Over the following days and weeks it became apparent that the violent activity we had been subjected to could be controlled by me channelling my energy into automatic writing. Whenever I felt that an attack might be imminent, I would sit down and let the automatic writing take over. With practice the messages became more coherent and intelligible, although in many examples their content was banal. The following is typical of the kinds of messages I received: 'John has got my spoons. Take them from him before he loses them. They are dear to me and they must not be lost. David Fraser, 1971.'

I became a magnet for the inconsequential musings of these entities, many of them seemingly deceased alcoholics or victims of car crashes wanting it to be known that they were not suffering or that their death had been quick and painless. I received messages with more substance once I began addressing questions to specific deceased individuals. I would put the name of the person I wished to communicate with at the top of my sheet of paper, and then write the question.

Of Bertrand Russell, I asked: 'Have your views on life after death changed since you died, or do you still believe that there is no life after death?' This is what came through:

Life returns on its way into a mist, its speed is its quietness again: existence of this world of things and men renews

ultimately their never needing to exist. Again knowledge will study others, wisdom is self-known and muscle masters brothers; self-mastery is bone; content may never need to borrow, ambition will wander blind, and as vitality cleaves to the marrow leaving death behind. The universe is deathless because having no infinite self it stays infinite. Clarity has been manifest in heaven and purity in the spirit. Man has no death to die. Bertrand Russell

The signatory at least knew how to spell Bertrand correctly. I had headed my paper with 'Bertram Russell', which I had mistakenly thought was his name.

After a while I was receiving as many messages in foreign languages as I was in English. French was the only foreign language of which I had some degree of knowledge, and it was very frustrating not to be able to understand what was coming through to me in Italian, German, Greek, Latin, Russian, Arabic and various Eastern languages, as well as Old English or Saxon. I would receive what appeared to be snatches or fragments of works.

One read like a series of French proverbs strung together: '*Je dis: aux grandes maux les grandes remèdes ou après la mort le medicin qui dit que la patience est un remède à tout maix. Marchand qui perd ne peut rire parce que les plus courtes folies sont les meillures.* Jacques Chaumont. 1933.' This translates as: 'I say: a desperate disease must have a desperate cure or after death comes the physician who says that patience is a plaster for all sores. Let him laugh that wins because the shortest follies are the best. Jacques Chaumont. 1933.'

Much of my summer holiday in 1971 was spent experimenting with automatic writing. One of my principal 'correspondents' was Robert Webbe, a previous owner of Queen's House, and the husband of the entity calling itself Anne Willis with whom I had communicated a few weeks earlier. I had compiled a mass of information on the Webbes during the winter of 1970 and spring of 1971 when I was engaged on an O Level history project for school. My original intention had been to write a history of the Webbe family, but when this proved impossible because large gaps in the information available from Cambridgeshire Public Records Office prevented me from being able to piece together a complete family tree, I decided to compile a history of the village of Linton instead.

Webbe made mention of this project in the first message I received from him through my hand: 'Your worke on our familye was most goode and very righte.'

This was the start of a mystery story that I would write as *The Strangers* in 1975. It seemed that Webbe had no idea he was dead. He behaved as though he was still the owner of Queen's House and his life was continuing, albeit after a painful fashion because of his gout. Much of the information that came through my hand from him was about his life as a gentleman. The following is the reply I received one night after I had asked him what he was doing:

'Indeed this very nite am I to have supper with mine goode man Rob: Moore and his goodley wife. She dost tickle myne fancey if I may say so.'

'What will you have for supper?'

'My good maide Beth doth prepare for us some fine bird with rabbit and sauce of blackberry and fyne wine.'

Queen's House had already been the scene of countless inexplicable occurrences, and contact with Robert Webbe instigated perhaps the most astonishing of them all during that summer.

On the morning of 31 July 1971 I found the name 'Rob. Webbe' written in pencil, in large letters, across one of the white-painted panels in my bedroom. As the walls were already dirty my parents decided it would be better to leave this piece of graffito rather than attempt to erase it. The three of us went into the garden to have a cup of coffee. Twenty minutes later my mother went back to my bedroom to look at the name. She found a second name – 'Hannah Webbe' – written in six-inch-high letters across another panel on the same wall. My father, when called by my mother to look at this addition, was not pleased. 'Tell Webbe that he is not to write on the walls,' he told me. I wrote my father's request on a piece of paper, and waited.

The reply was: 'Indeede I did see your owne fine workes on my familye and did decide to helpe you by allowing my frendes and allies to sign there names on the wall. You must realize that it is my wall and I am at liberty to write on my owne walls. Youre worke was moste fine and in moste part, very right.'

Between that day and 6 August over 600 signatures, the vast majority of them accompanied by a date, appeared on the walls of my bedroom. Many of the names were written in places where it was impossible for even the smallest hand to leave an inscription. Later I managed to trace many of the names in old parish records.

More than 200 signatures had appeared on the walls by the time my father invited a work colleague of his, William Nicholas, also an architect, to witness what was happening. The following is his memorandum of that visit:

Being a friend and professional colleague of Derek Manning, and having on numerous occasions expressed an interest in the extraordinary events surrounding his family, it was not without some inner feeling of excitement and expectancy that I set out to Linton early one afternoon. This visit was prompted by an invitation to witness with my own eyes the alleged culmination of several hours' hard work put in by some unknown agency. This agency was supposedly the erstwhile spirit/essence, energy or 'what-you-will' of one Robert Webbe, a former owner and resident of Queen's House, the destination of my visit. Robert Webbe had been selflessly employed in an apparently pointless task of collecting together a vast amount of signatures. These had been culled from persons long since deceased, and generously applied to various parts of the panelled wood surface.

Having hurried over, anxious not to miss anything, it was surprising to find the complete lack of excitement and utter calm which pervaded the house. They had all, of course, been living within the environment of the scientifically inexplicable, and therefore strange events, for years.

I was taken into Matthew's bedroom and shown the multitude of very interesting signatures which decorated the whole of one and a part of the other adjoining wall. These writings, executed with precision and care, using a black pencil, stood out clearly on the white-painted wall. Furthermore, Matthew had marked each and every appearance with coloured ink, thus recording date and order of arrival.

Having carefully examined the signatures I was accompanied by the entire household into the sunlit gardens, it being explained that the phenomenon did not and would not occur whilst the wall was under direct scrutiny. A pencil was left, however, hopefully on the bed. Some seven to ten minutes later we returned to find that another signature had been newly added.

This was then, and still is, one of the most interesting and mystifying direct experiences of my life. I am grateful that I was given the opportunity of being witness to this extraordinary event.

*   *   *

My parents decided to try to preserve the signatures as carefully as possible because they believed they were too valuable as evidence to be destroyed. However, by 1989 the room was desperately in need of redecoration and my father wrote to the Society for Psychical Research (SPR) to offer them the opportunity of making a permanent record for their archives so that he and my mother could at last redecorate the room.

The man given the task of photographing the signatures was

Dr Vernon Harrison, a graphologist as well as a professional photographer. He wrote an appraisal of the signatures and some of my automatic scripts and drawings, which was published by the SPR in October 1994. Harrison writes in his appraisal:

> One is struck by the profusion and variety of the writing. The size of signatures varies from more than two feet in length to down to minute inscriptions that require a magnifying glass to read. Signatures may be upright, sideways, oblique to left or right, and occasionally upside down. They are found from the skirting boards up to about eight and a half feet above floor level. One very large signature is scrawled on the ceiling. They are found on the mantel shelf and the window jambs. They are executed with a fluency and grace that are not only remarkable but in striking contrast to normal graffiti that I have been called upon to investigate from time to time.

On 3 August 1971 Webbe had written through me:

> I must explayne to you that I have not yet completed my many wordes. Do nothing for them still and I shall continue. Indede I did have no realisation of my many friends allies and familye. You must appreciate that I find it very difficult to do much work being somewhat infirm in bodily health. Some of these names are names I have written by me and methinks there are many more. I even knowe of half of a thousand such names. Some of them are people who have died on the place when 'twas that of the physik in 1363 and I knowe them not. I shall do my writing for three days more while you watch them before your eyes.

According to Harrison's analysis of the signatures, 85 per cent of them were written by Robert Webbe, 10 per cent by others; 5 per cent were 'capitals of dubious authorship', and nil could be attributed to my hand. He found that the range of the dates of the signatures was from 1355 to 1959, with 90 per cent of all dates falling between 1600 and 1855, and that '39 per cent of all signatures are dated after 1736, the year of Robert Webbe's death'.

Harrison found one of the automatic writings that I had taken down without premeditation of particular interest:

> I died in Switzerland on April 21, 1952. I am now restless. My body is at Sapperton. Where is Frith Hill? In the storm and uncertainty and fear that today permeate the world set yourselves to become part of the hand of God which stretches out to bring peace and patience and high standards of truth and justice to all peoples. Bless my body and allow mass. Here is Charles, father now. I must go.

I read the signature as Richard Cripps; beneath it was '52'. In fact, the signature read Stafford Cripps. Later I discovered that he was Chancellor of the Exchequer in the Labour Government after the Second World War. In 1950 he had been forced by ill health to retire from politics. He died in Switzerland on 21 April 1952, and was subsequently buried at Sapperton in Gloucestershire. He had lived at Frith Hill, and his father's name had been Charles. According to Harrison 'his signature is highly idiosyncratic and it is not well known. In fact I had difficulty in getting a genuine signature of Sir Stafford's for comparison.'

The Assistant Archivist at the Record Office of the House of Lords could find only one letter actually bearing his signature, written from the British Embassy in Moscow on 22 September 1941, addressed to Lord Beaverbrook. When he received a reproduction of the signature on this letter, Harrison writes:

> ... it shook me. The signature coming through Matthew is shaky by comparison with the confident one sent from Moscow, particularly at the beginning. It shows all the signs of a genuine signature made by a man suffering from old age, illness or stroke. It is not a copy or a forgery. If the signature in Plate 37 [the one that came through me]

were appended to a Will, providing that I had supporting
information about the testator's medical condition at the
time, I should have to pass the signature for probate as
genuine.

Of the handwriting of the message itself, Harrison describes it
as the 'most remarkable and interesting to come my way'. The
degeneration he noted in the Cripps script 'may have been due
to the sheer difficulty of controlling the medium's hand; and the
"anomalies" may arise from some form of interference from the
medium's brain and nervous system. I would expect there to be
some amount of distortion during the process of transmission.'

It was my mother who suggested that I should try automatic
drawing by attempting to contact a well-known artist and asking
him to draw something for me. The name she put forward was
that of Sir Alfred Munnings, the famous equestrian painter. Horses
are notoriously difficult subjects, and she knew that my limited
ability as a draughtsman would render it impossible for me to
draw one myself.

The drawing took an hour and when it was finally finished I
did not like the sinister, frightening image on the paper in front
of me. In the centre was a horse tied by the reins to a hollow-
looking dead tree. The backdrop to the main image was dead
grass in barren ground strewn with large hard stones. The sky
was a sweep of oppressive black clouds. Technically the horse
was the best thing in the picture.

That same day, I tried again, this time 'drawing' a camel, apparently under the guidance of Thomas Bewick. The camel was
technically better than the horse but, as with the automatic writing,
it seemed I was on a learning curve. The quality of the pencil
drawings improved over the following month, and I received
several more images from a variety of deceased artists. Some of
the drawings contained signatures, others did not. Among the signatures were the names of Paul Klee, Thomas Rowlandson and W.
Keble Martin. Later, drawings purportedly from Picasso, Beardsley,
Goya and Dürer would come through my hand.

One of the most baffling aspects of these automatic drawings was the wide variety of styles. My artistic ability had never excited interest and as myself I could not have reproduced the drawings that came through me. My school chaplain, the Rev. Treanor, confirmed this in a letter to Vernon Harrison:

> You may be interested to know that the school art department in Matthew's time did not consider that he possessed any artistic ability of his own. Moreover, there are teachers still present at Oakham who observed Matthew while he was drawing in a variety of styles. On no occasion was he ever seen by a member of staff copying from a book of illustrations.

According to my housemaster, Roger Blackmore:

> I can remember speaking to Matthew while he was doing some of the drawings and asking him how he felt about them. He could answer quite happily. He would talk about the period in which the drawing was based. He didn't appear to be in a trance. He was working as a normal artist of considerable talent would be working.

Most drawings are started by making an outline and then putting in the detail. Mine always started in the centre and moved outwards, complete in every detail as the drawing progressed. Interpretation was often not possible until the work was almost finished.

✳   ✳   ✳

In his analysis published in 1994 Vernon Harrison chose to comment in detail on two drawings purporting to come from, respectively, Albrecht Dürer and Aubrey Beardsley, both artists he much admires. The Dürer pen drawing was identified as a version of a portrait of Ulrich Varnbüler, the preparatory drawing for which is held in the Albertina, Vienna. A print from the woodcut derived from the drawing in the Albertina is to be found in the Department of Prints and Drawings at the British Museum.

After comparing my version with the print in the British Museum, Harrison concluded that mine was not a copy. The perspective was significantly different, as were the degree and style of detail in the drawing. My version was about half the size of the original Dürer. Harrison describes the portrait that came through me as 'a monumental tour de force'.

· Harrison found the drawing purported to be by Beardsley even more interesting than the Dürer. A pen drawing of a woman, satyr and peacock by a lake, it proved difficult to find its source. Eventually Harrison discovered that it is a composite of two drawings that were published around 1919 in a privately printed book, *Fifty Drawings by Aubrey Beardsley, Selected from the collection of Mr. H. S. Nichols*. In 1967 they were republished in *The Collected Drawings of Aubrey Beardsley*, by Bounty Books, New York. In the introduction to the latter edition, it is stated that the pictures from the Nichols Collection, 'are now deemed to be forgeries by the best authorities on Beardsley's work'.

The main arguments against the drawings in the Nichols Collection, apart from their faulty technique, are that 'they were twice as large as any known examples, that they were drawn on cardboard, which Beardsley never used, and finally – probably the most telling feature of all – that they were not included in Aymar Vallance's iconography which was revised by Aubrey Beardsley himself.'

I can still remember the feeling of frustration and irritation in my hand during the execution of my version. I was aware of mistakes being made and of them then being rectified by blacking out the offending area with ink and turning it into something completely different. I found out later that although he was a fine decorative artist, Beardsley was prone to making errors during the execution of his drawings. He had various means of covering these up – by scraping, by the application of Chinese white or, if the error was very bad, by sticking a fresh piece of paper down and drawing over it.

Harrison compared the drawing that came through me with the two forgeries. In all respects he considered the craftsmanship and style in the former as being characteristic of Beardsley. Many poor details in the forgeries seem to have been 'corrected' in my version. A badly drawn fountain in one of the forgeries has been eliminated in my version, and replaced with foliage and a small kiosk. In addition the general composition has been altered. However, my version appears to be unfinished, with a much larger than normal expanse of sky left unshaded. Harrison offers an intriguing explanation of this oddity and the others he has noted in the drawing:

> The differences between the forgeries and Matthew's version are not accidental. They do not arise by chance. They do not arise from faulty memories of a picture once seen but now largely forgotten. They are intentional, purposive. Wherever there is a difference, it is in the direction of better drawing in Matthew's version. These differences, which are tantamount to corrections, suggest that some intelligence has known about the forgeries and has sought to show us by practical demonstration just how faulty the drawing in them is.
>
> Aubrey Beardsley, if surviving in some form, might wish to do this when opportunity occurred. If the intelligence is not Beardsley, then who or what is it? Not, I am persuaded, Matthew Manning.

*   *   *

It quickly became apparent that the automatic drawing fulfilled the same function as the automatic writing in keeping the poltergeist activity in check. If I performed neither in a two-week period the activity would start up again. There was, however, a limit to my 'psychic' stamina. After about an hour I would begin to feel tired and the message or drawing I was receiving would lose clarity. I was shown a way round this as the winter term of 1972 drew to a close.

I had asked an artist purported to be Isaac Oliver to draw a picture of Queen Elizabeth I on a card measuring twenty-one inches by twenty-five inches. I knew this would take many hours to complete because every drawing that had come through my hand to date had taken up the complete area of the paper I was using.

The drawing was only partially complete when I was asked if, in its final form, it could be used to illustrate a school magazine. I agreed, not realizing that the deadline for inclusion was only a week away. When I was informed of this fact the day before the deadline, I knew I would have to disappoint them. A large area of card was still remaining to be filled and my reserves of energy were very low. I explained the situation to a school friend, who suggested that he round up a group of people and get them to concentrate on me while I continue with the drawing. In this way energy might be transferred to me.

His plan was worth a try, and with my agreement he went away to find four other willing minds. He and his group sat in a room about ten yards away and concentrated hard on me while simultaneously I concentrated on Isaac Oliver. Slowly, my hand began to move and my energy seemed to increase. After an hour and a half the drawing was finished. Many years later I would adapt this simple yet effective idea of generating energy and put it to a serious purpose.

It was in the winter of 1972/73 that George Owen suggested to my father that it would perhaps be interesting for me to have a reading with a clairvoyant. The only person Owen would recommend was Douglas Johnson, who had come to prominence in the Fifties and was well known in both the United States and Britain. My father went with me to Johnson's garden flat at Arundel Court in Chelsea, although he waited outside the room where the reading was held.

Johnson was in his mid-sixties, courteous and kind, and a completely different type from the man in Leicester. Almost as soon as we sat down together in his study it seemed he knew what he had to tell me. He did not fish for information or ask me probing questions about myself. What he said came out at amazing speed. The sheer normality of it struck me, as though I was listening to someone telling a story.

I have now forgotten much of that reading, but the snippets that have stuck in my mind have turned out to be accurate: 'Within a year you are going to write a bestselling book. There are going to be a number of connecting people in this but you are going to go to a very large mock Tudor house. It's white and it's got black beams on the front and there are two men living there. They are going to be pivotal to this book.'

At the end of the reading Johnson remarked, 'You will always have one foot in the stars and one foot in the shit'. His choice of language registered with me more strongly than any idea of what he might be trying to tell me! Later I was told that this corruption of Oscar Wilde's observation – 'We are all in the gutter but some of us are looking at the stars' – was a favourite of Johnson's and one which he applied to himself and those in whom he perceived a gift similar to his own.

My visit to Douglas Johnson coincided with my father buying a book entitled *Breakthrough: The Electronic Voice Phenomenon*. This was about the work of a Latvian scientist called Konstantin Raudive, who had managed to capture on tape what sounded like voices of the dead. I returned to school determined to try one of the experiments outlined in Raudive's book.

Late one evening five of us gathered in my study around a large tape recorder. We checked the tape to ensure that it was blank, ensured that the microphone was switched off, and then switched on the tape. We took it in turns to state our names and ask dead personalities to speak on the tape. Two fruitless attempts later we were close to admitting defeat and going off to bed, when one boy suggested that we invite Hitler to speak on the tape, reasoning that evil is always easier to summon up than good.

We switched the machine to record, and concentrated on Hitler's name for several minutes. Then we rewound the tape, turned the switch to the 'Play' position and waited. The gentle whir of the tape was broken by the deep rumble of distant artillery fire. This soon gave way to the uniform crunch of hundreds of booted feet moving in step. In the background we could hear the strains of a brass band playing a military march. The footsteps broke into a run as gunfire now accompanied the sound of the band. Incoherent shouting was audible too. Finally, there was the sound of running, echoing as though along a stone or concrete corridor. Then silence.

Raudive's book, however, offered more important guidance than I would derive from this experiment, fascinating and baffling though it was. Douglas Johnson's words kept coming back to me. The idea that I should write a book had not previously occurred to me, but now that it had been raised I wondered how it might be accomplished. My story was certainly unusual, possibly too unusual for many mainstream publishers, but then Raudive had managed to publish his extraordinary experiences. I looked at the copyright page of his book. The publisher was given as Colin Smythe, a name that meant nothing to me. Who would I write to there? I noticed that the introduction to the book had been written by someone called Peter Bander. Quite obviously, he was a man who could be trusted to take my story seriously.

Unbeknown to my parents, I decided to write to Peter Bander, care of Colin Smythe Limited, telling him that I had a story that might interest him. Almost by return of post I received an encouraging reply inviting me to telephone for an appointment, which I did from a phone box at school.

It seemed that both Peter Bander and Colin Smythe wanted to talk to me, and we arranged that I should drive down to see them in Gerrards Cross, in Buckinghamshire, on 27 May 1973, a Sunday. I had passed my driving test, and my father was happy to lend me the car when I told him that Smythe and Bander were interested in seeing examples of the automatic writing and drawing. I knew that if I told him the full story he would insist on coming too, and he would perhaps raise objections if the idea of my writing a book was mooted.

My father had endured years of reading end-of-term reports that exhorted me to try harder, apply myself to my studies and acquire genuine mental discipline. I had responded with brief bursts of determination. I had thoroughly enjoyed some of my school work, but I was not academic material. It was probably the automatic writing that made me realize how different I was from most other people. The questions crowding my consciousness could not be found in a book or answered by a well-tutored master. I was looking for answers to the inexplicable, and the content of many of my lessons seemed trivial in comparison.

My poor father must have thought he was home and dry. The offer of a place at Sussex University to study psychology was already mine. All I had to do was achieve decent grades in the A Levels in English and Sociology I was to sit in June and my future was assured. Instead I returned from Gerrards Cross clutching a contract, all thoughts of university gone, my mind set on writing the book Bander and Smythe wanted.

My father responded with great generosity of spirit when I told him what had happened and then asked for his advice. He said: 'I don't mind what you do so long as you're happy and you don't hurt anyone else,' which is probably the best advice that can be given to any child. If I wanted to write the book, I should sign the contract. He would support me for a year after I left school to enable me to write untroubled by thoughts of how I might keep myself. I signed the contract.

When I announced my decision at school my careers master reacted with disdain. He was sure I was condemning myself to a career of covering dog shows and fêtes for local newspapers. I was sure he was wrong. Underpinning youthful optimism was the memory of the image I had met on arriving in Gerrards Cross – a very large mock Tudor house with white-washed walls and black beams, and greeting me at the door the two men who lived there, Colin Smythe and Peter Bander. What I saw that morning exactly replicated the description given to me by Douglas Johnson.

Chapter 2

AROUND THE WORLD WITH MR JINX

O nly in later years have I appreciated the curious syn-
chronicities that brought me to the house in Gerrards
Cross. It had not occurred to me to write about my experiences
before I went to see Douglas Johnson, and how extraordinary it
was that my father should have bought Raudive's book, and I
should then have picked it up and got the idea to approach that
small, little-known publisher. When I first met Bander and Smythe
I had no book and no framework, but Peter Bander especially
could see the potential in my story and was probably responsible
for urging the more cautious Colin Smythe to take the plunge.

Initially there was talk about bringing in someone to help me,
someone with a sound reputation that would enhance the credibility of my story. One name put forward was Anita Gregory, a
well-known researcher and leading member of the Society for
Psychical Research. However, in the end it was decided that the
book would have greater impact if it was written by me alone.

My father gave me a £100 allowance to last for a year as well
as free board and lodging at home. I treated this money as a
loan, which I was determined should be repaid as soon as
possible. I did not want to be beholden to my father for anything.
(In fact, when the first royalty advance finally arrived – the sum
of £4,000, a small fortune to me then – my father threw on the
fire the cheque I handed him.)

We had assumed the book would take a year to complete. In
the event it took three months. I started writing as soon as I left
school in the summer of 1973 and during the course of those

three months was more often to be found in Gerrards Cross than at home in Linton. I had always been good at writing essays, and English was my best subject, so I was not daunted by what I had committed myself to, but I appreciated Peter Bander's help and advice, and we spent many hours working on the book together.

The project was given a provisional title, *Open to Suggestion*. Later I suggested *The Link*, the title under which the book would eventually be published, to reflect the notion of my experience representing a link between one reality and another.

Peter Bander and Colin Smythe inhabited a world I did not know existed. Their house was an education in itself, filled with amazing objects and paintings. I was used to being surrounded by antiques and quality furniture, but not of this highly deco-rated, showy kind. The house was large and was run with the help of staff, including a housekeeper. There was so much there for an impressionable eighteen-year-old to be impressed by. My father regarded it all with deep suspicion, especially Peter Bander, who came across to him as a self-opinionated waffler. My contract, though, was with Colin Smythe Limited, and Smythe himself had a reassuringly academic air and was quiet and cour-teous.

Bander and Smythe considered it important to introduce me to people with influence. Numerous dinner parties were given at Gerrards Cross for the purpose of making my name known among people who matter. Initially I regarded these occasions with awe and contributed little to them. I had to find my depth. Most of the people invited to Gerrards Cross were much older than me, and this was a greater inhibitor than the fact of them being established or well known in their respective fields.

Two of the first 'big names' I met were Fanny and Johnny Cradock, the TV super cooks of their day. She had a fascination for psychic phenomena and had been consulted by Peter Bander about the authenticity of a recipe purporting to be from Mrs Beeton that had come through me.

I also met the medium Doris Collins, who was as large and

intimidating as Fanny was over the top. Peter Sellers was one of her clients and she told us how he would ring her in the middle of the night to discuss his troubled relationship with Britt Ekland. Her stories about people I had previously only read about in newspapers were eye opening but did not make me relax in her company. I remember being very afraid of her and worrying throughout the evening about what she might be picking up from me psychically. I was too frightened to tell her what I was feeling and do not know whether she detected my unease. This experience has made me aware of some people's odd reactions to me in similar circumstances.

At the end of the three months it took to write *The Link* there was nothing for me to do except wait. Life at Linton was a bit flat after the excitement of creating the book and to-ing and fro-ing to Gerrards Cross. I just sat around all day doing nothing more constructive than firing my air rifle at tin cans. This seeming lack of application for weeks on end eventually chafed at my father's patience until one day he berated me for being a layabout who would not get anywhere in life. For the first time in my life I blasted straight back at him, and then walked out, vowing never to return. I went to Gerrards Cross and stayed there for about six weeks, until Peter Bander judged the time was right, on both sides, for me to go back to living principally at home.

That was the only real falling out I have had with my parents. From then on the relationship moved into a more mature phase and they relinquished control, accepting that I was now an adult and should be allowed to create my own life. When I got home I found flowers in my bedroom. My mother had never done this before and I took it as a sign that all was forgiven.

At the end of 1973 my attention was caught by the arrival in Britain of Uri Geller. Even at this early stage in his career, Geller was dogged by controversy and arguments raged over whether his astounding demonstrations of psychokinesis and mind-reading were genuine or whether he was merely a very good magician. In January 1974 my parents and I watched an ITV documentary called

Uri Geller: Is Seeing Believing? and after it my mother asked me if I would try to bend a metal object.

I was intrigued to find out whether I could emulate Geller. My mother handed me a stainless-steel spoon. I sat stroking the spoon and concentrating on it for about ten minutes. Nothing seemed to be happening to it, although I could feel something going out of my fingers. My father came into the room to see how I was getting on, and as I was talking to him I felt something happen to the handle of the spoon. When we looked at it we discovered that it had a kink in it and that it was continuing to bend, eventually to the point where it resembled the shape of a hairpin.

I was not absolutely sure that I had achieved this effect by means of psychic energy. My parents thought of a way of convincing me. My father gave me a six-inch nail, a quarter-inch thick, made of galvanized steel. I tried to bend it with my fingers, and when this failed I put it in a vice, also without success. I had proved to myself that I was incapable of bending the nail physically. Then I tried to influence it psychically, willing it to bend for some fifteen minutes. The nail remained resolutely straight.

By this time it was late in the evening and I was feeling tired. I decided to go to bed. As I was undressing I noticed that the large minute hand on the pendant watch I had been wearing around my neck was bent towards the glass. This convinced me that psychic force must have been in play at some point in the evening. I decided to put the nail under my pillow to see if anything would happen to it during the night. When I checked it the following morning, it had a bend in it of about thirty degrees.

I never derived satisfaction from metal bending, and considered it a fairly useless pastime. However, I did have one memorable experience when a man called John Steele asked me to 'test' a pair of handcuffs. The handcuffs he handed to me were not a common or garden variety. They were, he said, Clejuso handcuffs, one of the world's best – German made, of very special metal, unbendable yet lightweight.

It was a challenge I was not prepared to pass up at that time. I put on the handcuffs and wore them all that afternoon; try as I might nothing happened, and Peter Bander, who was guardian of the key, released me from them. Later in the evening, I tried the handcuffs again. At around ten o'clock, as I was watching television, I noticed that my wrists were feeling uncomfortable. Peter took the key and unlocked the right handcuff first. As the locking mechanism released and the handcuff opened, we realized that the ratcheted bar that secures the device was beginning to bend. When Peter tried the key in the left handcuff the mechanism would not budge. Clearly the two handcuffs had bent in unison.

Peter telephoned John Steele and explained what had happened. The question now was, how to get the left handcuff to open. Luckily Steele also lived in Gerrards Cross and it took him only a few minutes to reach us. He arrived in a state of high indignation, convinced that somehow we had got hold of the only machine in the world capable of bending his precious handcuffs. This machine was, apparently, a large, heavy apparatus, which it would have been extremely difficult to conceal.

Peter Bander invited Steele to search the house if that would make him feel any better. Steele then interrogated me for some time about what I had done. I had not done anything except to demonstrate that his Clejuso handcuffs were not impervious to psychokinesis. To cap Steele's indignation, Peter Bander succeeded in getting me out of the handcuff by sliding it off with the aid of washing-up liquid, albeit after a lot of difficulty and causing me some pain.

Steele went off, still fuming, and said that he would be sending the handcuffs to the police forensic laboratories at Brunel University for examination. The laboratory found that the right cuff had been bent approximately fifteen degrees and the left approximately ten degrees, and that no change in the molecular structure had occurred. Clejuso handcuffs are made of a base metal with a thin coating, which a deviation of only three degrees will cause to fracture. Special X-ray photographs of the handcuffs proved that the bends had not been produced by the application of physical force.

Presented with this evidence, Steele had to accept that physical means had not been used to get the better of his hand-cuffs. He would not, however, go one stage further and accept Brunel's findings as evidence of the existence of psychokinetic powers. 'I only know we are unable to explain in scientific terms what happened,' he would later tell the German magazine *Esotera*.

The episode with those handcuffs would come to symbolize my situation.

Shortly after completing *The Link* I was advised to sign a new contract, with Van Duren Publications, Bander's publishing outfit. This superceded the contract I had with Colin Smythe Limited, who were relinquishing copyright to Van Duren while remaining as pub-lishers. Peter Bander would take on the role of managing me while retaining his directorship in Colin Smythe Limited. Bander wanted to push ahead with publication as quickly as possible. I signed the new contract, confident that Peter Bander knew his way around this strange world of rights and opportunities.

It was decided that I should not take part in any prepublica-tion publicity for the book. Bander's decision was based on the media's ambiguous attitude towards Geller and the sometimes hostile treatment he was receiving. However, although I was in 'purdah' as far as the wider media was concerned, Bander care-fully prepared the ground for my eventual 'launch' on a largely unsuspecting public.

In his capacity as editor of a journal called *The Psychic Researcher & Spiritualist Gazette*, which shared premises with Colin Smythe Limited in Gerrards Cross, Bander primed his readership with stories about me and fed information to all corners of the small world of psychism and spiritualism in time for publication of the book. Bander had contacts with esoteric magazines in other countries, and articles based on me and my experiences appeared in these too. He was at pains to point out the differences between myself and Geller and not to highlight the similarities.

By dint of clever manipulation, Bander succeeded in whipping up interest among publishers while ostensibly keeping me under wraps. Several months before publication *The Bookseller*, the trade magazine of publishers and booksellers in Britain, was carrying snippets about the success Colin Smythe Limited were having in selling rights.

The conflicting publicity attracted by Uri Geller made me aware of the difficulties I might have to face once *The Link* was published. All around the world Uri was demonstrating his ability to bend metal. I could do that, and I could also do things that Uri could not. I was as unable to explain my powers as Geller was his, but that did not make me a fraud any more than it did him. The fact that the scientific community did not have a ready explanation either made it all too easy for the doubters.

I took the first opportunity that came my way to amass evidence in my favour that had the stamp of scientific authority. Out of the blue I received an invitation from George Owen to go to Toronto in June 1974 to participate in a series of experiments that were to form the basis of the first Canadian conference on psychokinesis, or PK – the effect that the mind can have on physical matter without physical involvement. Metal bending is a form of PK, as is the poltergeist phenomenon. The difference between the two activities is that the first is achieved consciously and voluntarily, while the latter is involuntary and outside conscious control.

The New Horizons Research Foundation, of which Owen was now Vice-president and Executive Director, had been founded – and was principally funded – by a weathy businessman, Donald C. Webster, with the aim of promoting research at the frontiers of science. This was a time of optimism in the field of parapsychology and it was hoped that the conference would represent a breakthrough in the understanding of psychokinesis. The delegates wanted to discuss psychokinesis in the light of actual experience of the phenomenon and needed someone like me to demonstrate forms of psychokinesis before their eyes. In short, I was there to give them something to talk about.

In March 1974 the Foundation had conducted a series of experiments with Uri Geller, which had been filmed live in the studio of CITY-TV in Toronto. Geller had caused a stir because in the bending and dividing of metal he was demonstrating a new form of psychokinesis. The scientists who took part in the Geller experiments were, according to George Owen, in 'no doubt that the objects – which were our own and recovered after the experiment – were bent or divided by some unknown process and not by common trickery'. The fact that I could also produce what they called the 'Geller effect' gave them a golden opportunity to take the experiments they had conducted with Uri one stage further.

During the ten days I spent in Toronto, from 18 to 28 June 1974, I bent or split between twenty or thirty objects. In the conference proceedings the types of key or cutlery and their serial numbers and makes are cited, the witnesses to each event listed, and first-hand testimonies given that I did not use any muscular effort to bend or, in some instances, split the objects given to me.

Even at this early stage I personally did not attach any significance to the activity of metal bending. It did not seem to prove anything other than that I could harness a destructive force. I particularly disliked the idea of that. However, if bending metal was what it would take to get scientists interested in finding an explanation for my unusual talents and helping me to understand me, I was prepared to go along with whatever they suggested.

One of the most interesting of the Toronto experiments for me was the one devised by psychiatrist Joel Whitton. He wanted to find out what, if anything, was going on in my brain while I was engaged in paranormal activity, such as bending metal. The measuring device used was an electro-encephalograph (EEG), which was attached to my scalp by means of electrodes. Our brain-wave patterns, which are made by the various levels of electrical activity in the brain, alter depending on what we are doing. My brain waves were measured while I was in various states: resting with eyes open; resting with eyes closed; making head, neck and eye movements; talking; and attempting to bend a key paranormally.

The experiment was conducted on several separate occasions, each time in the presence of various other conference participants. These included Professors Hynek (Chairman of the Department of Astronomy, Northwestern University, and Director of Dearborn and Lindheimer Observatories), Josephson (Cavendish Laboratory and Nobel Laureate) and Persinger (of the Psychophysiology Laboratory, Laurentian University) and Doctors Highman and Kurtz (both medical doctors). The results showed that the distribution of power in my EEG spectrum while I was attempting to bend a key paranormally was quite different from that exhibited while I was in any of the other states.

According to the report prepared by Professors Owen and Whitton, my EEG spectrum was:

> . . . characterized by a large concentration of energy in the Theta waveband (i.e. frequencies between 3 and 7 Hz.) and also by a linear relationship between the peaks in the Theta, Alpha (8–13 Hz.) and Beta ranges conferring a peculiar appearance on the graph of the power spectrum so that it was dubbed a 'ramp' function.
>
> The striking and unexpected nature of this result is best conveyed by noting that spectra of this kind with a major concentration of energy in the Theta band are only very rarely encountered in the waking state; instead they are characteristic of sleep in stage III or stage IV.

The next question for Joel Whitton was, 'Which part of the brain is producing this pattern?' Further tests with a computer at the Toronto Hospital for Sick Children revealed the source of the electrical energy as the limbic system, which lies beneath the cerebral cortex and may be described as the old animal brain we relied on before the development of our intellectual brain. Whitton concluded that the psychic power coming from it was 'not a random gift, but an innate function and ability in the brain of *Homo sapiens*, a function probably lost or defunct in most people for thousands of years'.

I was fascinated by the idea of my 'ramp function' being produced by the oldest, most central part of the brain. Intriguing too was the scientists' assertion that we use only 17 per cent of our brains. We can only imagine what is going on in the remaining 83 per cent. Whitton described the old brain as being able to 'think, feel and constantly does so, but not in a way it can put into words'.

What I use was probably something all of us called on at some point in our evolution, perhaps to enable us to find food, shelter, water or direction. For want of a better word, I shall call this 'intuition'. We have now largely lost it because to all intents and purposes we have no need of it – technological progress has seen to that. In cultures that live very close to nature (for example the Bushmen of the Kalahari Desert) intuition is an integral part of people's lives and it is widely used. It may be that every advance we have made technologically has added another layer to our intellectual brain, so that the gift residing in our limbic system is further removed from us. As we progress in one direction, we seem to regress in another.

A few days before the experiments with the EEG machine my electrical potential had undergone a different sort of measuring process when Professor Douglas Dean of Newark College of Engineering, a leading authority on Kirlian photography, took Kirlian photographs of my fingertips. The equipment he used for this was a Testa coil generator, or electronic leak tester, which gives about 25,000 volts alternating current at about 100,000 to 1,000,000 frequency in cycles per second with about 50 pulses per second. Radiation in the body shows up like a halo around the fingertips, and the Kirlian technique – named after its Russian inventor – renders the radiation visible.

Shots were taken of my fingertips with 'the power switched on' while I was undertaking paranormal activity, and with 'the power switched off' while I was in a normal relaxed state. Dean wrote afterwards:

In the resulting photograph the aureoles or coronas were much brighter for the 'powered' state than for the normal state. In addition, whiteness filled up the 'fingerprints' right into their centres, giving a cloud of brilliant white. I have never seen that before.

In further experiments Matthew was able to 'concentrate the power' into a narrow area and also to direct it into the middle finger only. In an experiment with two Kirlian devices, one for the right and the other for the left hand, which, by trial, were calibrated for approximate equality, he was able to make the power go into the right but not the left hand and vice versa.

Among the twenty-one scientists Owen had invited to the Toronto conference was physicist Professor Brian Josephson of the renowned Cavendish Laboratory and Fellow of Trinity College, Cambridge. In 1973 he had won a Nobel Prize for work he had done as a teenager while at university. Josephson had an interest in the paranormal and his approach to research was informed by his own experiences. He practised transcendental meditation, and many of his scientific discoveries had come to him either in dreams or while he was meditating. He noted that 'in physics there's the strange phenomenon that the laws of nature seem to keep on changing. New symmetry violations are being discovered, the velocity of light is found to be different from what people thought it was, and so on. . . . Perhaps one can modify the laws of nature.'

In Toronto Josephson tested my ability to deflect a compass needle. Before the experiment began I was searched for metal objects. The needle was at rest at the start of the experiment. When I passed my hand over the compass at a distance of about six inches the needle moved. The instant I removed my hand the needle stopped dead, according to the proceedings 'in spite of the fact that it was very weakly damped so that it would have been expected to continue swinging for some time'.

The reports of the Toronto experiments lent a huge amount of credibility to what I was doing. Without them I do not think

Colin Smythe Limited would have been able to pull off the publicity coup that ensured the success of *The Link* in Britain. The recently revamped *Daily Mail* agreed to run articles about me, based on the book, for three days, starting on 16 September 1974, before publication of *The Link* on 21 October.

The last of the three one-page articles, written by the paper's literary editor, Peter Lewis, caused a great deal of controversy. The topic of the article was 'the verdict [on me] of science's most respected names'. Lewis spoke to George Owen about the poltergeist effects and the automatic writing. He contacted Brian Josephson for his thoughts on the experiments in which he had taken part in Toronto. Josephson described to Lewis his experience while watching the needle during the experiment with the compass. He had 'felt a curious sensation in the eyes. It was as though I was seeing it through a heat haze, such as you get from a rising bonfire. When Matthew said his psychic energy was drained, my visual image suddenly became clearer.'

Josephson was describing what he felt, as you or I might. Scientists – particularly Nobel prizewinning ones! – do not usually talk in these terms. I recall Josephson being very excited by the Toronto experiments, as indeed were all the scientists who took part in them. Lewis must have caught him when he was still feeling upbeat and positive about the possibilites for further psychic research. He told Lewis: 'I think we are on the verge of discoveries that may be extremely important for physics. We are dealing with a new kind of energy. This force must be subject to laws. I believe ordinary methods of scientific investigation will tell us a lot about psychic phenomena. They are mysterious but they are no more mysterious than a lot of things in physics already.' When Lewis commented that in the past so-called respectable scientists would have nothing to do with psychic research and that many still would not, Josephson allegedly replied: 'I think the respectable scientists may find they have missed the boat.'

Josephson's remarks as quoted by Peter Lewis enhanced my reputation and gave me a solid platform from which to promote *The Link*. Josephson himself, however, came to regret them when broadsides were fired at him by his peers in the scientific community, and subsequently backtracked. Peter Lewis was adamant that he had captured Josephson's words on tape and what had been quoted was an accurate reflection of Josephson's views. Josephson labelled as 'inconclusive' the results of the test he did with me in Toronto, because he thought humidity in the room where the experiment took place could have affected the compass needle's behaviour.

This same experiment was later repeated by him at the Cavendish Laboratory in Cambridge, where the same effect on the needle was observed. When I 'switched on' my power the needle swung violently and equipment designed to measure changes in magnetic fields registered a change. When I 'switched off' the power the needle stopped dead. Professor Josephson could find no rational explanation for these occurrences, nor could he cite humidity as an influence on the results, yet he maintained that these results too were 'inconclusive'. His reaction constituted my first disappointment with the scientific community.

*   *   *

After 16 October 1974 my life would never be the same. This was my debut on national television. Through his extensive network of media contacts, Peter Bander had succeeded in getting me on *The Frost Interview* as the show's sole guest. It was probably fortunate that I had no idea just how 'big' this show was at the time.

I knew next to nothing about David Frost or his programme – the television ban at home in Linton was still holding. Only after a few people had reacted with horror when I told them the Frost show was to be my launch into the public arena did I become aware of what I might be in for. 'You must be crazy', 'He's dangerous', and 'He has politicians in tears' were just some of the comments that accompanied me in my first encounter with him a few days before the programme was scheduled to be shown. The impression he gave, however, was not of a man who was about to eat me alive and my initial nervousness quickly evaporated. He was easy to talk to and seemed genuinely interested in the story.

I came away from this meeting knowing roughly what had been planned to fill the show's forty minutes. A researcher called June MacFarlane had been brought in to organize the programme, to contact staff and former pupils at Oakham and to line up art experts to comment on the automatic drawings. All I was expected to do was arrive at the appointed time and follow David's cues. I knew nothing about how television programmes are made or what the inside of a studio looks like. I knew the show was going out live, but did not imagine this meant that almost 600 pairs of eyes would be trained on me in addition to the cameras. The shock of being confronted by that sea of faces when I walked out of the wings of the Collegiate Theatre towards where David was standing was considerable.

Shortly before that uncomfortable walk across the stage, I had been imagining that David might not be as nice as he appeared and that the Mr Hyde in his personality might introduce himself to me. The warm-up man had jokingly told the audience that I had a reputation for affecting electrical equipment, but that the BBC was an efficient organization and could handle any situation. He was referring to a recent incident concerning the products of a Dutch firm, Aura Electronics. This company had read about how, in Toronto, I had manipulated the energy of a Kirlian machine. Aura's Managing Director, Ted van der Veer, had asked if he could bring over to England the latest and most refined piece of Kirlian equipment for me to 'to put all the energy . . . [I] had into the machine.' At the end of the experiment, van der Veer had readily admitted:

> We can state categorically that the young man is able to produce an energy which cancels out 35,000 volts. At one point it appeared as if he was absorbing the entire 35,000 volts from the machine. The next moment he seemed to force an even stronger energy back into the machine

which caused it to break down....What we have seen is
simply incredible.

Problems of a similar kind began almost as soon as I sat down
in the chair opposite David. The engineers needed four takes to
get the show successfully underway. On the first take it was discovered that the equipment had not been recording. During the
second take a monitor that should have been switched off came
on. David noticed I was looking at it and said to the technicians:
'We only want that monitor on when slides are being shown. We
don't want it on all through the show. It's very distracting for
both of us.'

As they were setting up the third take, he whispered to me,
'Don't gaze at it.' Everyone was becoming a little nervous by this
time, including David himself.

On the third take David's first question to me was not picked
up on the tape. It was discovered that the sound was at half the
volume it should have been. The engineers insisted that the
volume setting had been correct at the start of the take.

'The return to Matthew Manning.' David quipped as we
waited for the countdown to the fourth take.

I am certain that the expectation of the audience that something might happen – an expectation excited by the throwaway
comment of the warm-up man – contributed to the technical
problems at the start of the show. Admittedly I was very nervous,
but that alone would not have been responsible for what
happened.

David had told me at our earlier meeting that he wanted me
to do some Thomas Penn diagnoses on the show. Thomas Penn
had made himself known to me one day in 1972 when I was
worrying about my grandmother. She was ill in hospital and
nobody seemed to know what was wrong with her. The following message had come through via automatic writing:
'Please may I take the liberty of asking the birth date of your
grandmother as it will help me. Do you consider the trouble
mental or physical?' I had written down her date of birth and

also that I believed her illness to be psychological in origin.

Penn's diagnosis turned out to be more or less what the hospital came up with. After this I was able to summon him at will. He only ever 'wrote' diagnoses for me and did not give any information about himself.

On *The Frost Interview* I was given the dates of birth of seven people in the audience who had specific health problems. I wrote down the dates in my handwriting and asked Penn to select one of them. He chose 12 August 1947. The diagnosis I wrote down was of someone with a back problem, a kidney malfunction and a history of heart trouble. The girl with that birth date confirmed the diagnosis.

A second diagnosis was received from Penn, for a woman whose birth date was given as 21 October 1947. David read out what Penn had written through me: 'Here basically we have a skin complaint. They suffer badly from a white blood corpuscle balance which is causing skin troubles and also affecting the lymphatic glands. There is a tendency of water in the legs. Strangely, at the same time we have a case of high blood pressure and brittle bones.'

The young woman whose birth date this was, said: 'I've got plenty of freckles but apart from that I don't think I've got any skin complaint. No, I've got a heart complaint. I've got malfunctioning valves.' She also denied having water in the legs.

I was asked to explain how it was that Thomas Penn could give one diagnosis that was spot on and another that was so wide of the mark. I said that, in my experience, Penn could get these diagnoses spectacularly wrong, but usually he was accurate. The second diagnosis was proved to be partially correct when the woman later admitted that she had a skin problem. However, it was proved to be correct in every detail when another person in the audience, who had exactly the same birth date, reported to the programme makers afterwards that she had all of the complaints described by Penn.

After the show everyone on the production side seemed very pleased with how it had gone. I was taken off to a prearranged party to unwind. I have only a vague recollection of that event, but I have never forgotten the drive to it with June MacFarlane. We were alone in the car apart from the driver, who could not hear our conversation. Almost out of the blue she said, 'Never forget that you have got where you are today in spite of Peter Bander, not because of him.' I was surprised by her remark and did not know how to reply. She changed the subject and did not allude to it again. I was to have reason to remember her words in the coming months.

The Frost Interview generated enormous media interest, although I was not aware of all the many offers of interviews and appearances that came my way. Peter Bander handled all enquiries and dealt with them as he saw fit. One request he turned down which I would have liked to accept was from Jean Shrimpton. The *Daily Mirror* had given several top models a camera and asked each of them to photograph the man she most admired. Jean Shrimpton had chosen me. Much to my disappointment, Peter Bander would have none of it, believing such publicity to be too downmarket. 'She'll be wanting to photograph you in your underwear,' was his comment.

Apart from effectively ending my anonymity, that *Frost Interview* changed perceptions of David Frost himself, probably for the better among the general public, but not among his own kind in the media, some of whom took the opportunity to attack him for devoting a whole forty-minute show to me. Frost had a reputation for being a very smooth, assured performer in front of the cameras, and on this occasion he had appeared flustered and sometimes lost for words, other than woolly ones, such as 'remarkable'.

There was a particularly critical review of the show by an up-and-coming journalist called Clive James, who was then television critic of the *Observer*. Frost's enemies had a field day raking over his 'weak' performance. The words 'rattled' and 'shaken' were used to describe him. Even the foreign press joined in – DAVID FROST REDUCED TO QUIVERING JELLY BY TEENAGE PSYCHIC was one headline in Australia.

I shall always be grateful to David Frost for being willing to run the gauntlet of ridicule. He is too astute not to have known what he was risking by interviewing me. I am not sure, though, whether he realized beforehand quite what a profound effect the events of that evening would have on him. I think they may have forced him to confront his own beliefs. This is a hard enough process for anyone to deal with in private, but to undergo it in front of millions of viewers must be so much more difficult, especially for someone who is expected to have an answer for everything.

The experience of the Frost show bolstered my confidence. I had found the tough man of television to have a very human side, so my next broadcasting engagement, on BBC radio's *Start the Week*, did not seem at all daunting. The format of the show was essentially relaxed conversation between people with unusual or interesting backgrounds hosted by a presenter. The role of the presenter was to draw out each contributor individually and then to encourage the other contributors to ask questions of that individual. On the programme that morning were its presenter Richard Baker, a Doctor Scott, Kenneth Robinson and me. Peter Bander and I had been under the impression that Dr Scott would be a psychologist who specialized in the paranormal aspects of psychology.

A few minutes before the programme was due to go on air, Dr Scott told us that he was Chief Statistician of the Bureau of Fertility of UNESCO; he had not read *The Link* and knew nothing about parapsychology. Apart from the presenter, this left Kenneth Robinson, who was a regular guest on the programme and, unbeknown to me, a somewhat controversial figure. Robinson had retitled the show 'Startle the Weak', a reflection of the delight he took in verbally beating up other contributors. He seems to have been famous for his biting wit. I do not recall much wit, only incandescent rage.

Perhaps Robinson's tirade of invective against me and the whole subject of the paranormal was no worse than his usual efforts, but the experience was very unpleasant. No one connected with the book was left unsavaged. Even the editor of the *Mail*, David English, was berated for having serialized it, and mimicked in a high-pitched voice. Robinson's ranting and raving were accompanied by almighty thumping on the table with his fists. Some Radio Four listeners thought that he must be physically assaulting me, and called the BBC to find out if I had been injured.

Afterwards Richard Baker apologized profusely for his colleague's behaviour. He would have ten more years of trying to mend the fences that Robinson purposely broke during the course of the programme, until Robinson was finally sacked. I was told that Robinson had been reluctant to appear on the programme at all, and had said that he did not want anything to do with 'that kind of thing'.

The fact that Robinson was a man of deep religious convictions may have been at the root of his antagonism towards me. I would come to learn that people who fear the unknown do react in this extreme way, and that the last thing they want is honest, reasoned discussion. It is always easier, and safer, to reject something that cannot be understood than to keep an open mind about it. Thinking afresh can produce a domino effect, and once a long-held belief system is questioned, other notions held to be dear or true also have to be re-examined.

I remember sitting in a traffic jam near Baker Street in London one day when a man suddenly stuck his head through the open window and started to shout abuse at me. He called me a charlatan, a fraudster and a hoaxer, and told me that I 'wouldn't get away with it,' whatever 'it' was. I found it hard enough dealing with pleasant people who came up to me in the street, never mind the ones who were downright rude. Eventually he wandered off, worn out by his exertions. It amazed me that he managed to summon up such anger so spontaneously. He could not have known he would come face to face with me on that particular day.

In general the press, especially in Britain, were enormously kind to me. The Toronto experiments helped to dampen their natural scepticism and encouraged the general public to accept

what must have seemed a very bizarre story. Even the quality
end of the press – from magazines to newspapers – did not
disdain to cover it.

The Link sold phenomenally well from day one of its publication. I was the least surprised of everyone connected with it,
apart from Peter Bander, who in the months before publication
had frequently rerun his vision of our future – 'It's going to be a
great story. I can see the newspapers jumping on us. A poltergeist
and a public school, and you've got the right voice.' My expectations were those of a naive seventeen year old. I thought that
if you had a book published it would automatically become a
bestseller. I had no idea of the thousands of books that do not
get published or of the thousands that do but never sell.

The Link was published simultaneously in Britain, Germany
and Holland, and rights deals were being pursued in other
markets. My immediate future was mapped out along a promotional trail of book signings, interviews, and radio and television
appearances. In Germany the book's success would, we were
told by publishers Verlag Hermann Bauer, largely depend on the
goodwill of Professor Hans Bender, Germany's leading psychical
researcher.

I was introduced to Bender at the book's launch in Germany
and it was arranged that I should take part in experiments with
him in Freiburg, where he taught at the University and was head
of the Institute of Parapsychology. These experiments were to
be funded by the German television company Süd Deutsche
Rundfunk (SDR), to whom Bender was already contracted for
several parapsychological programmes. In addition to taking part
in the experiments, I was to give an interview to SDR.

Bender was supposed to be in charge of how the experiments should be conducted and what should be filmed. However
this did not stop the director, Jorg Dattler, from trying to turn the
proceedings into 'good' television and urging me to perform
tricks instead of the experiments Bender had in mind. At the
press conference organized by Süd Deutsche Rundfunk, a
Professor Werner Schieberle from Ravensburg University had

brought along a gadget for me to influence for the assembled journalists. This gadget consisted of a power source to which were attached ten light bulbs on a horseshoe of wire.

The psychological pressure to 'perform' was as intense as the heat from the lighting for the cameras. I sat there for about fifteen minutes trying to get the bulbs to light up. After a final blast of concentration, two of them obliged. I was well pleased. The German media, though, were clearly disappointed in me. The headline in one of the newspapers the following day reported: PSYCHIC CAN ONLY LIGHT TWO LAMPS.

I was glad to leave this mentality behind and start work. In the first experiment I was asked to try to bend an opaque nylon tube through which a light beam was travelling. In one end of the tube was an electric light bulb, in the other a device to monitor the behaviour of the light beam. If I could bend the tube, the scientists reasoned, the monitoring device would immediately record a distortion of the light beam.

I placed my hands about ten centimetres above the tube and concentrated on it for several minutes. Nothing happened. Then I moved my right hand backwards and forwards, towards the end housing the light bulb. At this point the graph altered its tracing and began to register that the tube was bending significantly. The tube, however, showed no sign of this deviation and remained straight. In a later test with this piece of apparatus the monitoring device collapsed altogether.

The second experiment was with an electronic ESP tester, called an ESP-1AT. I had to predict the sequence in which the four lights controlled by the machine would flash on. The machine generates the lights randomly, so there is no danger of the subject of the experiment picking up telepathically from the experimenter the sequence in which the lights will come on. This machine failed after about ten tests, a situation which the machine's designer described as 'electronically impossible'.

These two experiments were conducted by two physicists from the University of Copenhagen, Professor Richard Mattuck and Scott Hill, who had been invited to participate by Bender.

The tests Professor Bender wanted me to do were entirely different in character. Bender was a psychologist who had already formed a pet theory about the origin of the phenomenon of automatically received information. He was convinced that the source was the individual receiver. A good test of his theory, he thought, would be to ask me to produce a drawing in the style of a completely unknown living artist of whom I had no knowledge whatsoever. He gave me a name, which I did not recognize, and told me that the artist in question was a woman.

After twenty minutes I had drawn a face of inexpressible sadness with a black heart set in its forehead, drooping eyes and down-turned mouth. Tears ran down its left cheek. On its otherwise bald head were two single hairs. Above these I had written the words 'Harliquin out of love'; incidentally, this spelling of 'harlequin' is incorrect in both English and German, and I have no explanation for it.

When Bender saw the drawing he demanded that the filming be stopped. He told us that the pseudonym he had given me was that of his daughter, who had been under a severe emotional strain since the breakdown of her marriage. That morning she had described her feelings to him and had used the word 'harlequin' to characterize them. According to Bender, in her psyche love and hatred had collided. He asked me to go with him to his house. A bigger shock was awaiting us there. We went in to the sitting room to find his daughter dressed in the costume of a harlequin, her face painted in a precise imitation of the drawing, her head shaved. She fixed me with an indescribable look, a mixture of sheer terror and intense hatred, before fleeing from the room.

Some twenty-five years later I still do not have an explanation for this happening. Given his daughter's unhappy state, it is likely that Bender's mind would have been filled with thoughts of her and it is possible I could have picked these up. But telepathy does not explain the self-mutilation of the shaven head or the exact replication of the mask she had painted on her face. Somehow I had tuned into her, not her father, although I had been completely unaware of her existence before Bender admitted the identity of the artist. Had she and I been involved in a parallel event, and while I was drawing the picture was she turning herself physically into the being she felt herself to be in her mind?

Psychological explanations of paranormal activity rely on established connections between individuals or foreknowledge, but none of these held good in this case. Unfortunately, Bender chose not to pursue the tantalizing questions the experiment posed. Out of consideration for Bender and his family, I agreed not to tell the full 'harlequin' story in public.

A few months after the experiment Bender himself gave an interview to the German magazine *Esotera*. He described 'Harliquin out of love' as 'a creative representation of something most complicated and paranormally received', a remarkable example of telepathy. He told only half the story, enabling his theory that all my automatic writings and drawings came from my own subconscious to remain unchallenged.

*   *   *

Some of the people who took an interest in what I was doing were not merely curious or students of the paranormal. Shortly before *The Link* was published I received what I thought at the time was an innocuous invitation to meet Lord Rothschild. According to a letter written by his wife to my father, he would value 'an opportunity to study the kind of phenomena that your son produces'.

Rothschild, a scientist by training, was on the brink of retiring from his job as head of the first Cabinet Office 'think tank', which had been set up by the then Prime Minister, Edward Heath. A couple of months after receiving this letter, I arranged to drive over to the Rothschilds' Cambridge home for a chat. When I got there I was shown into the study. It quickly became apparent that far from wanting to engage in stimulating conversation on the subject of psychic phenomena, Rothschild was after specific information. Our chat consisted of him grilling me for an hour about what I could do and what I could not do at a distance.

Would I be able to influence a piece of machinery? If I could influence a piece of machinery from a distance, would the effect diminish according to my distance away from it? Could I influence it more effectively if I was one metre away than if I was 500 metres away? Over what distance did I think telepathy could work? If someone was in the middle of the North Atlantic, would I be able to pick up what they were thinking? Did I think I could influence radar? Could I bring down a missile over the North Atlantic? If I was really angry with somebody, could I make their car crash? If I was close enough to the Prime Minister, could I read his mind?

I came away with the distinct impression that Rothschild had been embarrassed, which presumably he would not have been if he had been asking those questions on his own account. The general drift of his questions left me in no doubt that he was trying to find out if my powers might have military or espionage applications or possibly even security implications. I prayed that my answers had been so unhelpful and imprecise as to completely dispel the idea that I was some sort of one-man weapon system or nuclear deterrent. Our paths did not cross again, so we never did have our chat about psychic phenomena.

My suspicions about who Rothschild might have been helping out by making contact with me were proved correct years later. In the many obituaries and tributes to Rothschild on his death in 1990, mention was repeatedly made of his connections. An MI5 spy during the war, he had maintained his links with 'the firm', as that organization was known, and wielded considerable influence in the highest places until his death. He was said to have been regarded as 'the grand old man of espionage' and had been tapped for his knowledge and advice in this area by successive governments.

＊　＊　＊

Before the publication of *The Link* my experience of 'abroad' had consisted of two family holidays, the first in Holland, which I saw from the back seat of our Mini, and the second in Norway. My sense of wanderlust thrilled at the opportunity I was now being offered to see more of the world. Foreign publishers thought I could help generate sales, and wherever I went interviews, book signing sessions, and television and radio appearances were arranged.

I no longer remember many of the places I visited. They are points on a map that are as anonymous to me now as they were before I visited them. Their sameness reflected the uniformity of my experience with them. I was not there to seek out their distinctiveness, and the questions I was asked were the same whether I was in Amsterdam or Albuquerque. Of the many countries I visited during those hectic eighteen months of promotion, two made a lasting impression on me, and for very different reasons: the United States and Japan.

My first encounter with the American way came in the summer of 1975, when Peter and I embarked upon a coast-to-coast tour to promote *The Link* for US publishers Holt, Rinehart and Winston. The tour was arranged in cooperation with the *National Enquirer*, at four million copies America's biggest selling weekly paper, which was publishing weekly instalments from the book. On our itinerary were New York, Boston, Philadelphia, Pittsburgh, Chicago, Detroit, Minneapolis, Los Angeles, San Francisco and a few points between. No sooner would we touch down in one city than I would be whisked off to a radio or television studio, a bookstore or my hotel, where someone would be waiting, pen or tape recorder primed.

It was thrilling to be so much in demand, and the adrenaline was running for the whole three weeks. By the end of it, though, I understood why America is such a tough place. In the land of opportunity you are guilty until proven innocent, and this applies as much to new 'celebrities' as it does to people caught up in the legal system. I was probably naive to expect to be taken for an honest person.

Until this trip I had on the whole been treated gently by the media in other countries. In the States I found the finger of suspicion to be much longer and pointier than elsewhere, and the promotional ride much bumpier. I went there in a spirit of wariness, because Peter had given me some idea of what to expect. He handled the media on a day-to-day basis and was aware of attempts to put adverse spin on my behaviour or on what I had to say. Some people suspected me of being part of the so-called 'psychic circus' that had grown up since the appearance of Geller, and that I was 'in it for the money'. The truth was that the only payments that changed hands on my tours were strictly for expenses. I would not accept money for any of the dozens of appearances I made.

The same assumptions that had been made about Geller in terms of what he did were dusted down and applied to me. I too must be a trickster or magician of some kind whose particular brand of trickery would be uncovered in time. The American media were intent on exposing me as a fraud. I found myself being followed around the country and all my public appearances being scrutinized. Whatever I did, these people had an explanation for it. They wanted to prove that I was no better than they were.

On one live radio show, I had to guess what a person in the studio had drawn on a piece of paper. I have always been much better at transmitting telepathically than I am at receiving. When I am asked to receive, as on this occasion, I will ask the person to make a simple drawing and then telepathically communicate to that person what I want him or her to draw. I became aware of a man I had taken to be an engineer watching me very closely. He was in fact a magician from the Magic Circle, there with the producer's consent to make sure I was not using mirrors or watching the drawer's hand while the image was being executed.

Every time I turned up for a live performance on radio or television the American publishers had their fingers firmly crossed that I would cause some problem to excite further publicity. They were pleased when the sound system of the *Today Program*, broadcast from Philadelphia, went haywire for forty-five seconds on the morning of my interview with them, and delighted when, on a programme called *To Tell the Truth*, a spotlight above my head exploded.

The four celebrity panellists on *To Tell the Truth* had to decide which of three people presented to them was the real Matthew Manning. None of the panellists had read *The Link* or knew what I looked like, so all they had to go on was their intuition. The two others selected to pretend to be me were English schoolboys holidaying in the States. Each of us was introduced to the panel and asked a number of questions. The panel then voted, hope-fully matching the right person to the name. Just as I was being introduced to the panel as 'Matthew Manning Number Two' the spotlight exploded, sending glass everywhere and shattering the game of pretence. Up until this point only one of the four pan-ellists suspected that I might be me.

Underlying all my appearances on US television and radio was the pressure to 'perform'. Programme makers wanted to be sure that I could 'entertain' on cue. Because Uri Geller had 'dis-appointed' chat-show king Johnny Carson's expectations the year before, Carson had declined to have me on his show. Instead I appeared on the show hosted by Carson's chief rival, Mike Douglas. The actress Zsa Zsa Gabor was his first interviewee, and after he had finished talking to her and I came on she stayed and listened to what I had to say.

I suppose it was not surprising to ordinary viewers that this exotic Hungarian should have been interested in psychic phe-nomena. She could get away with not behaving like an American, not being one herself. What surprised Mike Douglas was her eulogy of David Frost's show, which she had seen on British TV. She kept on about how brilliant that show had been and how the Thomas Penn diagnoses had made her feel 'very spooky'. It was strange to have this ultra-glamorous creature – who obviously loved being the centre of attention – promoting me so heavily. For Mike Douglas's audience I gave a simple demonstration of telepathy, aided by a fellow guest, the singer Roger Miller. By the time Zsa Zsa had given her description of what had been served up on British television, this must have seemed very tame in comparison.

Sometimes book sales will be generated by the unlikeliest set of circumstances. Publishers will try their hardest to get you on a high-ranking TV show in the belief that sales will flow as soon as the closing titles roll. This undoubtedly worked in the UK with *The Frost Interview*, but in the States I had cause to be more grateful to a late-night interview with a little-known journalist called Jim Gallagher. He asked the usual questions, to which I gave my standard replies. He also enquired as to whether I had a girlfriend. I told him that I had not because at present I did not have time for one.

I recognized little from our chat when eventually I read his article. Subtly headlined HE'S NOT WASTING PSYCHIC ENERGY ON HIS SEX LIFE, it continued:

> 'I have no sex life,' says Matthew Manning, a nineteen-year-old British youth who says he's psychic. 'Perhaps this is where my psychic energy comes from. A lot of people think that psychic energy is connected with sex energy. I've come across a number of psychics, and I don't think that all that many are married. I think females are a pain in the neck. I don't like them and I don't date them. No, and I'm not gay either. I just have no sex life.'

I did not say any of this, but as the article in which this quote appeared was syndicated right across the States and it seemed to be helping sales, who was I to complain?

I came back from the States looking forward to a rest. After a fortnight of relaxing I was confronted by a headline on the front page of the mass-circulation weekly the *News of the World* (13 July) THE PSYCHIC AND THE MEN FROM THE VATICAN. The story, by Alan Whittaker, centred on two Vatican emissaries – Archbishop Hyginus Cardinale and Monsignor Bruno Heim – who were denying that they had consulted me about the then Pope's health. The *News of the World* reported that I had been given fifty birth dates for which I produced diagnoses over several weeks. Monsignor Heim was quoted as saying: 'It is true that Archbishop Cardinale and I met Matthew Manning, but we didn't consult him about the Pope's health. If you say so it would seriously embarrass me and I would have to deny it.' He admitted that a list of birth dates had been produced, but denied being the person who produced it: 'The whole thing was a very private matter and I am very concerned that it has come to your attention.'

I had been introduced to Bruno Heim by Peter Bander in 1975 and had on several occasions been to dinner at his Wimbledon home where I had met several Church leaders, both Anglican and Catholic. One of these was Archbishop Cardinale, Apostolic Delegate to Brussels who, like Heim, was a personal friend of Peter Bander's and was about to have a book published by him. I met both men again later at Peter's house in Gerrards Cross.

On this occasion I was asked to tune into a birth date to get a diagnosis of the person in question through automatic writing. It did not take too long for several sheets of paper to be filled with details of the anonymous person's health problems. The two men read them with interest and went into a lengthy discussion about the contents before explaining to me that the birth date in question was that of Pope Paul VI, who was unwell at the time with some mysterious illness his doctors were unable to identify.

I have never discovered whether or not the contents of the automatic script were correct or relevant, but later I received a thank you in the form of a beautiful papal medal bearing Paul VI's coat-of-arms, so I presume they were of help to someone. To this day the medal has a special place in my healing room.

The story in the *News of the World* must have sounded alarm bells of confusion and embarrassment in the Vatican. A few days after it appeared, the Vatican countered it through the *Catholic Herald* with the terse headline NO 'PSYCHIC CONSULTATION' –

ARCHBISHOP. Heim was quoted as saying: 'It is absolutely unthink-able that the Vatican should consult Matthew Manning or should give orders to consult him.' What is ironic about the denial of the *News of the World* story is that the Catholic Church is known to promote research into parapsychology. Perhaps, like science, it cannot be seen to have doubts about its own doctrines.

In public Peter was suitably indignant about the embarrassing situation his friends found themselves in. 'I'm incensed as you can imagine,' he told reporters. 'Bruno Heim is a friend of mine. Archbishop Cardinale has been a friend of mine for many years . . . Archbishop Heim and dear Archbishop Cardinale have been made scapegoats.' He also denied that there had been an 'official' consultation with me. The truth was that Peter had been respon-sible for 'leaking' the story in the first place. He had identified that 'private matter' as a fresh publicity opportunity and taken it.

By the turn of 1976 *The Link* was still selling in huge numbers and was being published in nineteen countries across the world (it went on to sell over a million copies). In November 1975 sales had been given new impetus by the publication of the book in a Corgi paperback edition. This launch meant another round of interviews and promotional work. The publicity strategy was working well: one appearance on BBC Television's *Nationwide*, hosted by Sue Lawley and Bob Wellings, catapulted sales from 2,000 copies in one week to 30,000 in the next. This time around the mass-market tabloids jumped on board. In an interview with the *Daily Mirror*, Paula James stated that I was 'as homely as bread and butter'. The content of our interview was summed up by the headline THE WEIRD WORLD OF MATTHEW MANNING.

A snappy headline is everything in the newspaper business, it seems, even a misleading one. The *Sun* contented itself with a brief review of the book under the headline THE EERIE WORLD OF MR JINX.

*   *   *

The strain of non-stop exposure to promotional work was worth it if one calculated it only in terms of numbers of books sold. I appreciated being able to afford an MGB sports car out of the proceeds, but it was my only extravagance. I was still living at home in Linton with my family, still enjoying the same small pleasures. The fame I could have done without, because people were as likely to insult me as to be nice. Of those who were nice, I could never be sure if they meant it and genuinely liked me or if they were only interested because I was in the public eye.

I had vowed never to sell any of my abilities, for example by predicting winning horses or the rise and fall of share prices. Once, though, out of sheer devilment, I did let my 'halo' slip. I had gone into a pub with a friend, who then decided to play the one-arm bandit machine in the corner of the bar. He was not doing very well so I gave him a hand. During the course of the evening we succeeded in emptying the machine twelve times. The publican asked us not to come again unless we promised to leave his machine alone.

In January 1976 I set off for another series of laboratory experiments, this time in Sweden, principally with Dr Nils-Olof Jacobson and Jan Fjellander of the Forsknings-center för Psykobiofysik in Stockholm. A psychiatrist by training, Jacobson was well known in Sweden as the author of a book on the evidence for survival after death. Fjellander, a social anthropologist, had overall responsibility for conducting the experiments. The weekly magazine *Hemmets Journal* was sponsoring the experiments as well as paying my expenses. In return the magazine expected to have exclusive coverage of the proceedings in the laboratory and of the results later. It was also arranged that I would spend five days doing experiments with physicist Georg Wikman at the Chalmers Tekniska Institut in Gothenburg.

Wikman had devised an electrostatic meter, which I was to attempt to influence. I sat in a chair in a room whose floor, ceilings and walls were lined with aluminium foil. Eighteen measurements of the electrostatic field were taken at intervals of thirty seconds. When we were about two-thirds of the way through these measurements, the graph jumped from 2.1 to 9.2. Wikman noted: '. . . when this happened Matthew was holding his hands in the air and not moving his feet . . . Whether this was a "paranormal" effect or not could not be *concluded* [his italics] but the facts point in this direction.'

Thomas Penn diagnoses formed the basis of the first experiment in Stockholm. Jacobson presented me with a list of ten birth dates that corresponded to ten patients selected at random from the records of a general hospital. I was asked to give a Thomas Penn diagnosis for each patient. The names of the patients were written on the same piece of paper, and I found it difficult not to let my concentration wander from the name on which I was supposed to be focusing to the others. After the experiment the Penn diagnoses, together with shortened case histories compiled by Jacobson, were to be passed to medical people not involved in the experiment whose job it was to match the diagnoses to the appropriate case histories.

Another novel experiment was a seed-growing test devised by Jacobson. One of the early pioneer researchers into psychic healing, itself a kind of psychokinesis, was Dr Bernard Grad of Montreal's McGill University. He became interested in this area after meeting the Hungarian healer Oscar Estebany in the late 1950s. One of the experiments in which these two collaborated was a test with barley seeds watered with salt solution. Each experiment showed that the plants watered with saline that Estebany had treated – simply by holding in his hands the bottle containing the saline solution – were, to a statistically significant degree, the more rapidly growing ones.

In the Jacobson experiment there were three test tubes, each containing a grass seed. Jacobson knew the rate at which these seeds would grow if they were kept under controlled and identical conditions. With one tube I was to concentrate on energizing the seeds positively to make them flourish; and with the second to concentrate on energizing them negatively, to retard their growth. I was to leave the third tube alone. A scientist who had not been involved in the first part of the experiment took the tubes away to transfer their contents to trays. The tube marked 'A' would be transferred to the tray marked 'A', and so on. The results of the test would not be known until the seeds had grown and the treatment each tray had received was revealed.

The final experiment was very similar to the nylon tube test I had done with Richard Mattuck and Scott Hill in Freiburg. The apparatus consisted of one metal 'house' containing a transformer, fuse and 12-watt light bulb, and a second containing a photosensitive resistor, with a 9-volt DC circuit. The light beam was projected through a thick cardboard tube. The metal 'houses' and the tube were joined together to ensure that the beam could not be interfered with physically. My task was to try to influence the beam. I could not see it, so I tried to imagine my hand passing through it.

After a short time a furious clicking noise could be heard coming from the direction of the 'house' containing the light bulb; the sound was very like what had often accompanied poltergeist activity at home and in school. A V-shaped bulge then appeared in the otherwise perfectly straight moving graph band, which was monitoring the beam. According to this reading the light beam had suffered severe distortion.

The scientists decided to make a control run. At this point, in Fjellander's words, 'the device started to behave very strange', and seemed to absorb a large amount of energy. The clicking noise started up again, this time accompanied by a loud hum. The physicists and electrical engineers eventually traced it to the electrical circuit and the 9-volt DC battery. This puzzled them because such a hum can only occur in a current that is in constant flux between AC and DC. Our device was not running from an AC current, such as the main electrical supply, so how could this be happening? They were still searching for an explanation when a fuse blew and the whole apparatus went dead.

The scientists stripped down the device, found nothing untoward – apart from the blown fuse – and put it back together again. The experiment was rerun, with the same result – I concentrated and the fuse blew. The third try was just as unlucky.

After that the scientists gave up. When I pushed them for explanations, they could give none.

I came home from Sweden wondering what had been achieved. It seemed that I was caught in a trap scientists had made for themselves. The laws of physics could not be used as a yardstick to measure non-physical energy, and yet here they were applying them. New laws would have to be developed if any progress could be made in psychic research. But where were the scientists to devise these laws, to challenge orthodoxy, as Einstein had Newton?

I told Peter that I did not want to do further experiments on physical phenomena. We agreed that in future the scientists would have to convince me that what they had in mind was worthwhile and that they were committed to getting a result, and not simply repeating the same experiments to achieve the same 'inconclusive' results.

I was tiring, too, of the promotional treadmill, of being constantly at the beck and call of foreign publishers, and having my words vetted and channelled. Wherever we were, Peter Bander seemed to speak the language. That was useful so far as getting around and ordering food were concerned, but as a way of life it was personally undermining. I was beginning to feel like a prized commodity and not a human being with his own identity. I had got used to Peter taking over interviews and deciding what should be attributed to me. For months I had been telling myself that most of the questions were so predictable and boring that he might as well answer them as me. And yet. When he decided not to accompany me to Spain, where I was to spend eight days visiting Madrid, Barcelona and Valencia to promote *The Link*, I was secretly pleased. He was as fed up with the travelling as I was, it seemed, and sent his assistant, Leslie Hayward, in his place.

In addition to doing interviews and book signings while I was in Spain, I took part in a telepathy experiment with Professor Ramos and seventy-eight of his students at Madrid University. I made a drawing that I tried to communicate telepathically in order for them to reproduce it. I chose to draw a circle with rays emanating from it. Seventeen out of the seventy-eight reproduced the drawing exactly; thirteen drew a circle minus the rays; and some others produced drawings that were neither right nor completely wrong. Ramos was pleased with the result, which was well beyond the bounds of probability.

Unfortunately, Uri Geller had been in Madrid the week before and had managed to stop the escalator in a department store. The one question asked by just about every Spanish journalist who interviewed me was: 'What can you do?' One of my least favourite topics of conversation at this time was Uri Geller. Wherever I went it seemed he had been there a few days earlier. This would not have mattered if I had been less anxious about my status in relation to his but, like some insecure prima donna, I was fed up seeing his name in headlines more often than mine. The competitiveness between us shot to unimagined heights one evening when I went to do a signing session in a large department store.

The people crowding around me urged me to 'do' something. I did not want to oblige. I was there to sign books, and so far as I was concerned that was it. The atmosphere changed when the people who were pressing me realized I was not to be swayed. Frustrated by my refusal, they started jeering at me. This insulting attitude made me furious. I was on the verge of letting them know this when, suddenly, the lights went out and everything powered by electricity stopped functioning. It was assumed there had been a power cut until it was realized that other shops and premises in the street had not been affected.

Emergency generators had to be used while the store's electricians hunted for the source of the failure. Eventually the power was restored, but the technicians could not find a fault anywhere in the electrical supply system. I am convinced that the cause of the problem was the people themselves, and not me. They wanted something to happen and it had. This was my first experience of the power of a collective will. Four months later I would be at the centre of an even more spectacular – and frightening – example of the same phenomenon.

The opportunity to visit Japan was offered to me by a Japanese psychic researcher, Toshiya Nakaoka, who asked me if I would appear on a live ninety-minute television show called *Wednesday Special*. Japan was a country I had always wanted to know more about, so I asked if, in return for appearing on the programme, I could be shown some of what remained of the old Japan. The new Japan was all too evident when I arrived in Tokyo on 28 June, a modern miracle of economic progress, boasting every consumer durable known to mankind. I wanted to step back and experience the country as it had once been, before it was opened up to Western influences.

Nakaoka and an interpreter took me by bullet train from Tokyo to Kyoto, Japan's capital from AD 794 until 1868, when the Emperor Meiji was restored to the imperial throne with an agenda to modernize. I loved Kyoto, with its magnificent art treasures, its ancient Buddhist temples, its long tradition of learning. Everything that makes the heart of a nation beat was here, I thought. In the surrounding countryside I saw people living as they had done since time immemorial, quietly, simply and in harmony with nature.

While I was in Kyoto I did some automatic drawing and writing which were filmed for the forthcoming programme. The most interesting of these was a message that was later identified by the priest of the Daikaku Ji Temple as an example of Bonji, an ancient Japanese script once used by the monks of that temple. Daikaku Ji was one of many temples I visited, and one of the oldest. A site of meditation for centuries, it seemed an appropriate place in which to receive an impression from the past.

After five days we 'bulleted' back to Tokyo. I felt like someone with the 'bends' who returns to the surface of the sea too quickly after a period of immersion in its depths. We began work on the programme. It had already been agreed with Nakaoka that I should demonstrate automatic writing and drawing in addition to giving a lengthy interview to the programme's presenters. The show's producers were hoping for something more spectacular to keep the audience's interest for ninety minutes. They were banking on me producing the same effect as Uri Geller had when he appeared on Japanese television. The station involved had been deluged with calls from viewers, so twenty-five telephone lines were installed in a studio adjacent to the one in which I would be working for the duration of the programme.

As the day of the transmission crept closer I became aware of increasing nervousness among the production team. Perhaps they were worried about the programme turning out to be a damp squib and their ratings falling. When we went on air they were not encouraged by my showing the contents of a box filled with items that had appeared at Linton over the years: these included a rock-hard bread roll, a fish-shaped snuff box, some beads and a leaf fossil.

One of the presenters, Kiyoshi Kodama, said, 'Oh, that didn't really happen, did it?' A couple of minutes later a note of a call that had come through was passed to Kiyoshi. A woman who lived at the other end of the country said that she had been watching the programme when a large glass ashtray that was sitting on a table in front of the television set had inexplicably split in half with a loud bang.

Kiyoshi decided to call the woman to get her to reiterate her story for the benefit of the other viewers. He got a wrong number and spent several minutes at cross purposes with the person at the other end of the line. Eventually he got through to the woman, who described her experience. While Kiyoshi was talking to her all twenty-five lines in the other studio were jammed with calls from hysterical viewers. Several hundred individual stories were noted down from the 1,200 or so calls received that evening.

A company executive, Taizo Öno, living in Ömiya-shi Saitama-ken, said that he and seven eyewitnesses had seen a packet of cigarettes split in half, as if it had been cut with a knife.

A Mr Baba, an assistant professor of electronics at the University of Technology in Toyko, said that he had watched an

eighty by ninety centimetre painting on the wall above his television set swing like a pendulum and then turn a complete circle.

An unprecedented wave of poltergeist activity swept across
Japan. There were many reports of glasses, bottles and objects
shattering for no reason; fluorescent lights exploded; watches
were affected: broken ones started working again, and functioning ones stopped; taps turned themselves on; electricity was
switched off; ceiling lights and lamps changed colour from white
to red; stuffed birds and monkeys disappeared; things material-
ized – cigarettes, coins, dolls, even a boiled egg; a long-lost ring
returned itself to its owner and was found on the table in front
of the television set; several colour televisions would only receive
in black and white, and some owners of black and white sets
were treated to colour; a cupful of coffee went solid; boiling
water poured into a vacuum flask turned into ice; car engines
were turned on without keys in their ignition; one person found
10,000 yen on his sofa; the alarm system of a bank called the
police out, stopped when they got there, and started up again
after they left.

The Japanese are very organized, and the producers had
taken the precaution of compiling a minute-by-minute schedule
for the entirety of the programme. This was abandoned and
Kiyoshi and his co-presenter, Yoko Nogiwa, went excitedly with
the flow. Stories were coming in of interference to rival channels,
whereas NET, the channel putting out *Wednesday Special,* was
unaffected. There were reports too of some televisions deciding
what their owners should be watching, and switching from other
channels to NET. Such unilateral moves helped to boost ratings
to 27 per cent, some 3 per cent more than the previous all-
channel record, and 17 per cent more than the programme
usually achieved.

I was as amazed as everyone else by what happened. When
I had a chance to think about it, amazement gave way to
depression. People were regarding me with awe, but they were
missing the point. I may have opened a door but *they* had been
instrumental in creating the mayhem of that evening. Although

a range of poltergeist activity occurred, the vast majority of the incidents involved the splitting or shattering of glass in people's homes.

I think it is no coincidence that of all the many countries I visited Japan was the only one in which this poltergeist activity occurred. The Japanese are relatively conformist in how they dress and behave, and rather excitable, too. To my mind this adds up to a sort of assembly-line personality, like cars that are essentially the same apart from differences in minor details such as colour and accessories. The Japanese seem to me to have more of a 'herd consciousness' than other nationalities. It is interesting that the poltergeist activity occurred right across Japan, reflecting perhaps a common unconscious response. To what, I am not sure. Perhaps it was tacit acknowledgement of a national psyche split between materialistic wants and spiritual needs.

I returned home from the thirteen-day trip exhausted, and similarly split between my wants and needs. Japan made me face myself and a growing disenchantment with my life. I knew I could not carry on as before, performing tricks to no good purpose, like some organ-grinder's monkey. If I carried on in the same way, what would my legacy consist of? A heap of broken computers that people could not work with, and a pile of bent spoons that people could no longer eat with. In short, I would have done nothing useful. I had to find something practical to which my gift could be applied.

My decision to stop and take some time out to think about my future was not greeted with enthusiasm or understanding by Peter Bander. He had not been in Japan with me. As in Spain, his absence had allowed me the psychological space I needed to form my own impressions and to make my own decisions as to how I should react to people and situations. Looking back, it was not surprising that he should have greeted my news so coolly. I was the proverbial goose laying large golden eggs. Peter tried to talk me round, and because I had no wish to upset him I agreed to the proposal he put to me. I would write a second book to capitalize on the success of *The Link*.

For months Peter had been dropping hints in interviews about a controversial book on which I was supposedly working, which he called *A Shot in the Dark* – ironically and, I think, coincidentally, the name of a film in which Peter Sellers starred as the farcically inept Inspector Clouseau. Bander was hopeful that some gullible publisher would take the bait and swallow his long line about the book's 'explosive' contents. I thought there was insufficient material to justify what he had in mind and urged him instead to publish a typescript I had already completed, about Robert Webbe and the extraordinary haunting of my parents' house.

This was too dull a proposition for Bander, however, and he insisted that we stick to his plan. He told me that I was now an established name and he had brokered a deal for UK rights with W.H. Allen, a London publishing house with a much higher profile than Colin Smythe Limited. W.H. Allen wanted someone to work on the typescript with me, to give it a style that was, to their way of thinking, more appropriate to the large 'market' they envisaged being out there waiting for my next offering. The book, retitled *In the Minds of Millions*, turned out to be what it had always promised, a triumph of style over substance, the exact reverse of *The Link*.

For months I worked half-heartedly on the book, between honouring promotional commitments and thinking about what I should do next. One of the magical things about youth is being able to believe in life's possibilities. A young person may not even be able to name one of these, but he or she knows it is out there, somewhere.

In 1976 this idealism was fostered by the example of the hippy movement, albeit somewhat crinkling at the edges by now. At school many of my friends had older brothers or sisters who had at least flirted with hippydom, and a lot of the music I liked was of that era. In the early 1970s it was very trendy to go out to India and find a guru or mystic who would sit cross-legged on the ground and give you the answers to life. I planned to take the same path, to go to India and find someone who could give me direction. This would be my next goal after I finished the book.

* * *

I arrived in India on 27 March 1977 and stayed there for the best part of four weeks, travelling around to find this all-knowing man who would give me the answers to life. I followed all the tips I was given on the road as to who this guru was and where he might be found.

India itself was a culture shock like no other (not even Japan) and it opened my eyes to the meaning of poverty. I had never imagined, let alone seen, such appalling living conditions. I saw a man riding through the traffic on a bicycle with a dead body wrapped in a shroud. An everyday occurrence, I had to conclude, because no one else seemed surprised. Lepers on skateboard-type vehicles would bang their stumps on the windows of my taxi. My immediate reaction was to give money to anyone who looked in need. This was not an answer, because as soon as I did so I was engulfed by people wanting the same. I could not single-handedly provide for India's poor.

I remember leaving Delhi early one morning and as we were driving along coming across a group of people sitting on their haunches at the side of the road. It was obvious that something had been hit. I was getting used to seeing all sorts of animals dead or bleeding in the road, left for the vultures. To start with I thought the victim was a cow, but as we got closer I realized it was a person. His top half was on one side of the road and his legs were on the other. None of the people was doing anything. They were just sitting around and watching. I found this very hard to understand.

Shortly afterwards I went down with food poisoning. I had been warned not to drink the water, and to eat only fruit that I could peel. I even brushed my teeth in Coca-Cola to avoid drinking the water. One day I was so thirsty I bought a bottle of

Coke from a street vendor who was keeping the bottles under ice
in a bucket of water. I drank from the bottle, and that was it –
diarrhoea and vomiting for days. It struck while I was in a taxi
miles from anywhere. I had to keep asking the driver to pull
over. We would stop in what appeared to be some vast, empty
plain and within a couple of minutes there would be Indians
everywhere, hanging out of the trees, appearing out of drains.
They were there, it seemed, just to watch me. One of my lasting
impressions of India is of its swarming, curious people, everywhere.

The experience of being constantly exposed to what I considered appalling snapshots of life went in at a very deep level.
I began to hate the country, and I became really cynical about
not being able to find a guru and the reason for it. Probably
there were no gurus left in India because they were all sitting in
luxurious air-conditioned chalets in Switzerland.

I spent my last week of the trip fulfilling a childhood ambition
– to see the Himalayas. I hired a car with a driver from Delhi
and headed north-west to the province of Himachal Pradesh. As
we climbed the foothills we passed wizened sherpas, carrying
great tea chests on their backs, symbols of the leisurely pace of
life in this rural area. We passed through the region's sprawling
capital, Simla, a famous hill station in the days of the British Raj,
and onwards towards Tibet. The road deteriorated quite
markedly after Simla but I decided that we should push on to
Narkanda, a distance of about forty miles. My one fear was that
we might be involved in an accident. There were no restraining
rails on the mountain road, which in places was barely wide
enough to allow one car to pass. When I looked down I could
see sheer drops, thousands of feet deep. If we came to grief, we
would never be found.

Our only casualty was the car, which broke down suddenly
almost as soon as we reached Narkanda. The scenery was so
spectacular, I did not mind in the least. I had no idea how high
up we were – only about 9,000 feet I discovered when I looked
at a map, although it seemed as though were looking at the top

of the world. All around us and rising up steeply were the jagged peaks of vast mountains.

My knowledge of mechanics being precisely zero, I could not offer the driver any helpful suggestions. I left him to sort out the problem and made for a rock some forty feet away, intent on taking in the awesome surroundings. I reached my objective barely able to breath. The reason for the car's sudden reluctance to go further clicked in my brain: the engine could not cope with the thinner oxygen at this altitude.

It was now late afternoon. Darkness would soon be falling. I decided that we should stay the night and arranged accommodation for myself in what was euphemistically called a guest house. The driver slept in the car. I doubt that he was less deprived of creature comforts than I was that night. My room was jumping with bugs, and the en-suite facilities consisted of a stinking hole in the floor. Chary about eating what was on offer, I had obtained a couple of fresh eggs, which I intended to prepare myself. I lit a fire in the grate in my room and when it had died down placed them in the hot ashes to cook. They repaid my ingenuity by exploding. It was the coldest night I have ever spent – even Oakham had been cosier than this. I got no sleep and spent the time planning what I would do the following day.

My first objective was to get up before dawn to position my camera on a tripod. I had a very good Olympus camera with me and I wanted to take one of those arty California type photos of the sun breaking behind the mountains. I set up my camera and waited. I did not take that photograph.

As I watched the sun rise something happened which to this day I have difficulty describing. Suddenly, and I do not know whether it was for one minute, one second or ten minutes, because I lost all sense of time, I felt completely at one with and connected to everything around me. I became a part of the mountains and the rocks. They were part of me. I was the air, the air was me. I was part of the tree and the tree was part of me.

In those timeless moments of transcendence I came as close to God as I am likely to get on this earth. I was aware of a presence urging me to do only what I felt was right and what I wanted to do and not what others wanted me to do for their own reasons. I must also follow only those paths that would lead to healing. This last prompting struck me as very strange. I knew a little about the sort of healing given by people such as Harry Edwards but had taken only a passing interest in it. I interpreted 'healing' in its broadest sense and took it to mean more than putting my hands on people.

I left India a few days later, grateful for all I had experienced. Even the appalling poverty and suffering seemed to have meaning now and became fused in my memory with that revelation in the mountains. No guru could have taught me more. The irony was that had I received the same wisdom from a teacher, I would not have listened. That is my nature. I always have to experience or know something for myself, and go with my intuition. None of us needs a guru to point the way. The route is mapped out within us, although too often we are either sidetracked by the influence of others, or internal static and white noise drown out that inner voice. I had heard mine loud and clear and knew I could move forward.

Chapter 3

NO FAITH
REQUIRED

The experience in India taught me that everything in the
universe is connected in some way. Whatever we do has
implications for somebody or something else and filters through
to other levels of existence. The chaos that had ensued from my
appearances in Spain and Japan had made me look hard at what
I was doing and acknowledge the destructive potential in psychic
energy. I wanted none of that. What intrigued me was the idea
that my thoughts might be able to affect the metabolism of an
organism. If this notion could be proved under laboratory conditions, good might come of it.

In late 1976 I had made arrangements to take part in experiments with scientists in the United States. This had been made
possible by a man called John Evans, who had approached me
after becoming aware of my interest in doing this kind of work.
He had a good friend at the University of California, Professor
David Deamer, a zoologist, and through him arranged for me to
spend three weeks with scientists at the University's Davis
campus, which is situated just outside San Francisco, and a
further ten days with researchers at the Washington Research
Center in San Francisco itself.

A few weeks after being contacted by John Evans, I received
another invitation from the States, this time to speak at a series of
conferences on self-development and spiritual awareness. Public
speaking was a completely new area for me and one I was keen
to try. Two years spent plugging *The Link* around the world and
doing countless talk shows had smoothed the corners off my

shyness. Financially the offer was very attractive: $500 per day for one hour's lecture plus air fares and other expenses. The conferences, scheduled to start in June, would also neatly fit around the series of experiments which were to begin at Davis soon after my arrival there.

My ideas on the kinds of research work I would like to be involved in had come sharply into focus after India. I regarded the forthcoming trip to California as a great opportunity to do experiments that might one day benefit people. Before I arrived, I asked if the scientists would bear this in mind when devising their tests. On the evening of 18 May I met all the participants at the home of Doctor Fred Lorenz to discuss their plans. Lorenz, who was Professor Emeritus of the Department of Animal Physiology at Davis, proposed several tests that had positive applications.

For our first collaboration, Lorenz put a novel spin on an exercise which is routinely done in school laboratories to show how sodium ions are transported across the skin in frogs. This transport is effected by a nerve impulse (axon), an electrical phenomenon whose changes in activity can be recorded by attaching electrodes to the skin. In laboratory experiments tactile stimulation is applied to the nerve to record the impulse. Lorenz wanted me to try to mentally influence the nerve. This experiment seemed to me to have potential significance for cases of paralysis because, if successful, it would show that nerves could be made to work other than by the usual physiological mechanisms.

Working with separate pieces of skin, I and the control subject, Dave Deamer, attempted first to increase and then to decrease the active transport current by holding our hands a few inches from the membrane and sending out psychic energy. I imagined that I was holding the original frog from whom the skin had been taken and sending a terrific surge of healing energy through its body, restoring it to life. According to Lorenz:

When Matthew attempted to increase the active transport there was no change in the already high value of 125
micro amps in one minute, followed by an increase of 8
micro amps in 20 seconds and then a gradual decrease
back to the original level.

MM's attempt to decrease the active transport rate was
cleaner and much more dramatic. Immediately after he
started work the current started to fall and decreased
from 80 to 40 micro amps in 10 seconds. This low level
was maintained for a little over a minute and thereafter
the current increased somewhat irregularly in spite of his
continued effort, but had not regained its original level
at the end of the run.

In contrast, DD's attempts had no effect on the active
transport current.

One of the most satisfying aspects of the experiments in
California was the willingness of the researchers to take into
account some of the human issues involved in experiments with
psychokinetic energy. These were especially apparent in a series
of tests in which my task was to attempt to influence people psychically, by either sedating or arousing them. The measure of
my success in this activity was electro-encephalography, or EEG,
as for the previous experiments in Toronto.

EEG is normally used to monitor the electrical activity of the
brain in the detection of disorders such as epilepsy and brain
tumours. Normal brain waves are known as alpha waves and
occur with a frequency of about ten per second. Abnormal waves
are known as delta waves and occur with a frequency of seven
or less per second. Lorenz wanted to use EEG to assess the level
and nature of the 'brain waves' occurring in me and in subject
individuals during periods of influence.

Fred Lorenz was keen to be my first subject. He was seated
in an isolation room with eyes closed while I sat outside. Both
of us had electrodes attached to our scalps, and the leads from
these were plugged into a device that 'traced' the information

picked up by each electrode. The pattern created by all the traces shows the state of the brain and the level of consciousness of the individual to whom the electrodes are attached.

As Lorenz was part of the experiment, the task of experimenter was given to Professor Loring Chapman, who was Chairman of the Behavioral Biology Department of the Medical School at Davis. I received instructions from him to arouse or sedate Lorenz, or to rest. A clear result was achieved, according to the traces and Lorenz's own recollection of what happened. He was:

> ...very aware of being alerted three times, with drowsy or inattentive periods between.... My first remembered alerting was most dramatic and seemed to come out of deep drowsiness or even actual sleep.
>
> The correspondences between MM's [EEG] and my own were most dramatic. These are most clearly illustrated by moments such as those where trains of high amplitude or slow waves are simultaneously evident from both heads. Especially interesting was a kappa rhythm which manifested simultaneously in both heads. The kappa rhythm is usually a sign of alerting during a drowsy state.
>
> The correspondence was not limited to such short-term and striking displays, however. It seemed that usually when Matthew was producing alpha rhythm, so was I. There were three consecutive pages of an awakened period; i.e., they cover 30 seconds of record. During that half-minute MM's record and mine shifted simultaneously (though not with the precision of some of the patterns already described) from low amplitude, fast beta to irregular, slow waves and then to quite regular alpha. Such correspondences could be seen throughout the record.

When the same test was subsequently tried with two different subjects, no apparent correlations were recorded. These results are intriguing because my experience of these individuals was strikingly different. The first of them, Barbara, had been specially invited because of her previous successful participation in unpublished experiments with Lorenz. These had involved simultaneous EEG records of two subjects making psychic contact. Lorenz was hoping that she and I would be able to make similar contact for him to explore.

Unfortunately, we did not click and, worse, I felt that she was resisting my influence to arouse or sedate her. Certainly the EEG records did not show that she was responding to my efforts. Next morning Lorenz suggested that we try the experiment again. The atmosphere seemed all wrong to me and I felt unable to attempt it. Instead it was agreed that we should focus on a neutral object. During this test I became uncomfortably aware of the electrodes and the holder-cap on my head, a feeling that intensified as the experiment went on. We were getting nowhere, as the EEG record showed, and eventually it was decided to stop.

I put this apparent failure down to the negative feelings that Barbara evoked in me and suggested to Fred that we try the experiment with another subject. Shortly before I left Davis for San Francisco, we reran the trial with a girl called Cindy. I had built a rapport with her and was confident that a personality clash would not compromise the test this time. Almost as soon as we began the experiment the discomfort I had previously experienced with the electrodes returned. Cindy's experience paralleled my own, and she reported that the electrodes suddenly caused her a lot of pain just before the run started. Our EEG traces did not reflect these effects, but my guess is that Cindy was psychically picking up or resonating with my discomfort.

I learned a great deal about the nature of my psychic ability during the time I spent in California. One conclusion I reached was that maybe it has its own in-built boredom threshold. In three sessions of tests conducted by Professor John Jungerman, in which my task was to attempt to influence a machine which generates random numbers, 'significant' results were obtained only during the first session and my scoring significantly declined over the three sessions. (To a scientist the word 'significant' means that the possibility of an event occurring by chance is very low and that there is a high probability that the variable being tested – in all these experiments, me – is causing the event to occur.) Science demands that tests should be repeated over and over again to prove their validity. Perhaps in psychokinetic terms, once is enough.

All but one of the experiments in extrasensory perception were conducted at the Washington Research Center in San Francisco, with either James Hickman or Doctor Jeffrey Mishlove. The most successful of this series involved my identifying which of ten sealed canisters contained water. Uri Geller had already demonstrated his ability to do this (with researchers Targ and Puthoff, 1973) so, naturally, I was game to see if I could match him. Ten opaque 35-mm film canisters with tight-fitting lids were selected by Hickman. While I waited in a separate room one of these was partially filled with water and then all ten canisters were placed in a random sequence on a table.

My ability to pick out the right canister seemed to improve over the three days the sessions were held. The first session consisted of two runs. In each run I had ten attempts to select the correct canister. I chose correctly once out of the first ten attempts and twice out of the second ten attempts. By the fourth session, I chose correctly eight times out of ten attempts in both runs.

At my suggestion, an additional run of ten attempts was conducted, this time with a ball bearing replacing the water. Again I chose correctly eight times. I learned during this experiment to trust the strong impulse I received sometimes as soon as I saw the canisters. When this impulse occurred, I chose correctly. Sometimes I would perceive a faint field around a canister and frequently this denoted the correct canister, but sometimes it did not. When I relied on pure guesswork, I usually got it wrong.

In another ESP experiment Mishlove selected four 'target' illustrations, sealed them in manila envelopes and handed them to an assistant who brought them to me in a separate room.

Mishlove did not enter the room I was in during the experiment to guard against the possibility of my gleaning subliminal clues from him. I was asked to psychically guess what these illustrations were.

Mishlove had excluded from this target pool an image that he thought might trigger negative emotions in me because it showed the abusive ways in which some scientific researchers have been known to treat their subjects! Somehow I must have picked up on this because elements from the rejected picture were evident in all my responses to the four target images. Although the results of the test were not that great, they provided strong evidence of ESP displacement and the operation of an uncontrolled form of psychokinesis in my responses.

This displacement effect was also evident in a coin-spinner experiment conducted with Charles Tart and John Palmer at Davis. My task was to make a spinning silver dollar fall either 'heads' or 'tails'. The spinning was done mechanically by a machine fitted with a plexiglass shield and a shock-absorbing mechanism to prevent any breaths or bodily movements affecting its coin-spinning apparatus. I completed three runs, each one consisting of fifty trials.

Before my visit Tart and Palmer had discovered that the machine showed a consistent 'tails' bias and so in the trials with me had alternated target faces. 'Heads' had been my target for the first run, 'tails' for the second and 'heads' again for the third. Also, for the first and third runs the coin had been placed in the holder with the 'heads' side up and in the second run 'tails' up. Five weeks after I left Davis, according to Tart and Palmer's report:

> To our surprise, we discovered in retrospect that the coin showed an overall heads bias during the three runs where Matthew was trying to influence it. The number of heads on these runs were 31, 25, and 28, respectively, for a total of 84 heads, a 56 per cent heads bias, exactly opposite the 55.6 per cent tails bias we had in control runs.

In an ESP feedback-training test conducted at the same time as the coin-spinner experiment, I produced another unexpected psychokinetic result, this time with ADEPT, a machine designed for training forced choice ESP. I found ADEPT rather irritating, and derived pleasure in causing it, in Tart and Palmer's words, 'an enormous variety of transient malfunctions, consistent with a poltergeist type of manifestation'.

I had given no interviews while I was at Davis but as soon as I moved down to San Francisco a number were arranged, principally to advertise a forthcoming appearance at the Marin Civic Center, San Rafael – billed as 'an intimate evening of discussion with Britain's celebrated young psychic' – which was to be hosted by Dr Stanley Krippner, the world-famous parapsychologist. Krippner had made his name in dream research when, as Director of Maimonides Dream Laboratory in New York, he had devised pioneering experiments into sleep and telepathy and published his findings in a highly readable book, *Dream Telepathy*.

According to Krippner, we are at our most telepathically receptive during sleep, and our dreams can be influenced by another person concentrating on a particular image or thought. He asked his friends in the rock band The Grateful Dead to help him with one experiment which, perhaps because of their involvement, would become his most famous. Krippner wanted to show that the number of people concentrating on an image could vary the influence on the sleeping person.

The band members were interested in his research and agreed to allow an image to be projected on to huge screens at the back of the stage while they were playing a live concert in California. The idea was that the tens of thousands of people in the audience would 'send' the image telepathically to a sleeper at the Maimonides Laboratory. The result of this experiment supported Krippner's suspicion that the greater the number of people concentrating, the greater is the influence on the sleeper.

Since Maimonides, Krippner had moved on to become a faculty member at the Humanistic Psychology Institute, an educational body concerned with 'the higher possibilities for human development'. Krippner saw these 'possibilities' as involving ordinary people in making greater use of their own unrecognized and undeveloped subconscious gifts. He and I shared a common interest in finding ways of applying these gifts to the practical advantage of society. During the evening at the Marin Center we discussed a range of ideas, including the establishment of holistic medical groups and centres where people could learn how to develop their potential, and setting up a group of psychic researchers. Our discussion was followed by me sending the audience three telepathic images. Judging from their response, this appeared to be moderately successful.

In his introduction to the evening, Krippner had asked everyone in the 850-strong audience to note the contents of their belongings and to report any changes. Shortly before the end of the evening, he asked if anything unusual had occurred, but no one volunteered any information. As he was leaving the auditorium Krippner looked at his watch, which was indicating 10.20 p.m. He was pleased because this meant he would be home by 11 p.m., in time to see a favourite television programme. When he arrived home the clock in his kitchen was indicating midnight. He was puzzled as well as disappointed. He remembered checking the time at 8.10 p.m., when the event began. He knew that the watch was well wound and had rarely given trouble since he bought it twelve years previously.

A few miles away Jack Kerolis, the co-producer of the Marin event, was equally puzzled. On unpacking the contents of his briefcase he had found a printed page that he had not seen before. Kerolis knew that the leather folder in which he found it had at the start of the evening contained only a pad of note-paper. He was certain, too, that the folder had not left his hands at any time. The page contained information about Human Dimensions Institute West, a personal-growth oriented organization in Southern California. Kerolis had heard about this organization but this was the first time he had seen any of its literature. A short time later he would be introduced to the director of the Institute, Lucio Gatto, and discover that Gatto had attended my evening talk with copies of that printed page in his briefcase.

✳   ✳   ✳

Stanley Krippner was particularly interested in cross-cultural approaches to the practice of healing; he had co-authored a book called *The Realms of Healing*. His research had brought him into contact with a remarkable Native American medicine man, Rolling Thunder, a revered man who had an awesome reputation as a healer in the States.

I was amazed when, a few days after our appearance together in Marin County, Stan told me that Rolling Thunder had asked him whether it would be possible to meet me. Rolling Thunder had, it seemed, been aware of me since my first trip to the States to promote *The Link*. I could not believe my good fortune. A meeting was arranged to coincide with a time when Rolling Thunder would be staying near San Francisco, at the ranch of musician Mickey Hart, drummer in the super-group The Grateful Dead. Stan had told me that both Hart and the band's guitarist, Jerry Garcia, were very interested in exploring the possibilities with automatic music.

The mental picture I had of Rolling Thunder and the reality could not have been more different. I suppose I was expecting an impressively tall, strong chieftain in buckskins and full head-dress. The only evidence of the ancestry of the diminutive, greying figure that greeted me was his face. This was weather-worn and etched with lines which seemed to radiate out from a pair of deep-set, sparkling eyes. He wore a battered check tweed suit with the trouser legs untidily pushed into wellington boots.

Stan, Hart and fellow Grateful Dead band members Donna and Keith Godchaux and Jerry Garcia were at the ranch the evening I met Rolling Thunder. It became apparent as soon as the introductions were made that Rolling Thunder viewed me with a mixture of curiosity and wariness. I thought it best to let him take his time assessing me rather than try to force conversation on him, and concentrated on talking to the others. Garcia and Hart were very interested to see whether I could make automatic music. After all, if I could do it with writing and drawing, why not with music?

Hart invited me to try and sat me down at his piano. At this point Rolling Thunder became very disturbed and insisted that everyone stand in a ring around me, holding hands, while he blessed the air with a feather. This ceremony had no positive effect on my attempt at the piano. Hart wondered whether I might do better with a guitar, but the results with that were equally dire.

When I got round to talking to Rolling Thunder I found him fascinating. He told me that understanding begins with respect for the Great Spirit. What he called the Great Spirit, I had called oneness or interconnectedness since my experience in India. He believed that many of the people seeking spiritual guidance were looking only for something that would benefit themselves. The ego, he said, had to be transcended before one could become spiritual.

Thoughts of giving healing at some point in the future had been in my mind for months. Rolling Thunder raised my awareness of what it entails far beyond my limited concept that it would involve closing my eyes and putting my hands on people. He told me about his way of working, which is in a tradition that medicine men from his culture have followed for thousands of years. Native American medicine embraces all of nature and teaches the individual to find harmony with it. The ideal is to become connected with the spirit and all of life. When this occurs the body, as well as the emotions, mind and spirit, are healed. According to this philosophy, medicine is anything that allows us to step into our personal power and strength.

The Native Americans see life as a circle within which we move from birth to death to rebirth. At birth we enter what they call the medicine wheel and thereafter pass through the wheel's four quadrants. Each point of the wheel is akin to the four seasons in nature and represents a different direction and a different element, and has different qualities assigned to it. In psychological terms, for example, each quadrant represents a different aspect of our personality; Jung, it seems, was not breaking new ground by coming up with the idea of the personality having four aspects. If we get out of step during our journey around the wheel, we risk illness.

Rolling Thunder explained the principles of the four elements: air, water, fire and earth. All the elements, he said, have their source in the spirit world and it is by acknowledging them that he and other medicine men are able to gain wisdom, power and mastery. If I was to practise healing, I must understand the origin of the energy with which I was working. Ignorance might allow evil spirits to work through me. I should learn how to protect myself from such influences and respect the forces. Communication with the elements would then be open to me, enabling me to become a part of nature and not an antagonist or victim of it. He imparted the following to me:

- In nature, **air** circulates high above the land and has an overview of life. The part of us that has air has the ability to see far. It is illumination, integration, creativity, and is the universal part of us.
- **Water** is the feminine part of our being and represents feelings and emotions. It is intuition, our deepest connection with spirituality, our sacred dreams, psychic impressions and inner knowing.
- **Fire** is the power of transformation, because it purifies and renews, changing old patterns and old habits. It represents the alchemy that occurs when we release the old and embrace the new.
- **Earth** is wisdom and grounding and enables us to stand firm in times of adversity. It is health and the food we eat. In nature, earth is trees and plants, rocks and stones, as well as the ground we see.

When Rolling Thunder finished telling me this, I realized why he had been slightly ill at ease on first meeting me. He had been concerned that evil spirits might be working through me and had wanted to ensure his own protection and mine – hence the brief ceremony at the piano.

At the end of our conversation, Rolling Thunder stood up and asked us all to go outside with him so that he could perform a healing ceremony and give me spiritual protection. He had, it seemed, suspected I would be in need of protection even before he had set eyes on me. We followed him to a clearing surrounded by trees, in the centre of which he had collected wood for a fire. He told us to collect stones, which we were to use to make a perimeter circle around the fire but a few feet from it.

When the circle of stones had been laid, four cardinal stones, representing the four elements, were placed on the ground pointing north, south, east and west. Rolling Thunder then offered a prayer to the Great Spirit to ask for a blessing during the ceremony into which we about to be initiated. He smudged each of us with ash from some grass he had burned, to purify or consecrate us. The fire was lit and we stood ready to enter the representation of the medicine wheel, the one pathway to peace, harmony and integration of the self.

Each of us had to close our eyes and take seven deep breaths before entering the circle from the east. I felt myself relax and connect with the air as the wind breezed across my face and I became aware of my breathing. I moved around the circle to face south. Rolling Thunder had positioned the cardinal stone at this point so that when standing by it one was caught by the sight of the sun glinting off the surface of a nearby lake. He told me to focus on the water and to feel its energy. At the western cardinal stone I faced the fire and drew in its energy. Then I moved around to the northern stone to connect with the energy of the earth.

In each quadrant of the circle Rolling Thunder asked us individually to sense the qualities of the element, to assess how those qualities related to us, and to feel a part of that element. With only the quiet, deep voice of Rolling Thunder breaking the silence, we all moved close together in the centre of the circle. I could feel the energies spiralling towards the middle. The medicine wheel was now complete. Rolling Thunder told us to send up our prayers to the Great Spirit in the knowledge that they would be answered.

The whole ceremony took over an hour and at the end of it I was in a state of wonder. I had not realized how powerful and energizing such an exercise could be – probably for the simple reason that I had never before stilled myself for an extended period to become aligned with the elements. The experience was empowering and yet soothing, and for some time after the ceremony I wanted to remain quiet and attuned to the connections I had made.

The principles of this ceremony have remained with me ever since that incredible night. I would never see trees, rocks, water or any of the elements in the same light again – all hold their own energies that infuse the totality of life. On a personal level, whenever I am tired or drained of energy, I return to them to restore my inner balance. Professionally, they would inform many of my attitudes and show me that there are many different, yet equally valid, ways of healing.

I felt that everyone present was affected in a similar way, and had been shifted into a different state of awareness. From my first meeting with Mickey Hart I appreciated that he did not fit the stereotype of a rock star I had held in my imagination. The other band members were similarly easy-going, intelligent, sensitive people who revealed themselves to be genuinely interested in issues beyond the narrow sphere of rock stardom. One of their ongoing projects was to support Rolling Thunder's tribe, the Shoshone, by raising money through charity concerts.

At this time the band were in the midst of recording the album *Terrapin Station*, and a couple of days after our meeting they went into the studio to record a song by Donna Godchaux called 'Sunrise'. The song is a tribute to Rolling Thunder and a reminder that the wheel is never ending and is, like nature itself, a constant process of renewal.

*   *   *

The last of the California experiments was conducted on the day before my departure, with James Hickman at the Washington Research Center. It was a repeat of the grass seed test I had done with Professor Jacobson in Sweden the previous year. Although eighteen months later I was still awaiting written confirmation of the success of that experiment, I was confident of its validity and wanted to try it again. Of all the series of experiments I was undertaking in California, that one seemed the most useful.

Hickman filled three vials with commercial rye grass seeds, sealed them and labelled them A, B and C. He gave me vial A with the instruction to try to increase the normal yield. I held the vial for five minutes, all the while closing my eyes and concentrating on encouraging the seeds to grow. I was asked to decrease the growth of the seeds in vial B. I held the vial in my hands, closed my eyes and this time concentrated on retarding the growth of the seeds. Vial C was not given to me. A colleague of Hickman's transferred the contents of all three vials to new vials, coded Q, T and W, and locked the key to these codes in a safe until after the statistics were completed.

On days nine, ten and eleven after planting, Hickman counted the number of sprouts and measured each plant. The total height and quality of all the plants whose seeds I had encouraged to grow were observed to be significantly greater than those in the control group, the original vial C. The plants whose seeds had been in original vial B – whose growth I had tried to retard – were not as tall as those originally from vial A but taller than those from the control group.

The California researchers took a refreshingly different line to the spontaneous occurrences that happened around me as a matter of course. Most of the researchers I had worked with before had either ignored or rejected them on the grounds that they had not occurred under controlled conditions. This argument has always amused me – in anybody's language a spontaneous occurrence is by definition uncontrolled – and seemed to be yet another example of scientists refusing to

contemplate anything that does not fit neatly into their limited –
and limiting – perameters.

The report published by the Washington Research Center
includes anecdotal accounts of spontaneous incidents that may
have involved psychokinetic energy. Many of these incidents
were reported by the researchers themselves or other people
associated with me during my stay. One of the most intriguing
involved a research assistant, identified in the report as RA.

On returning to her normal research activities a week after my
departure, RA began to experience a series of inexplicable
computer breakdowns. A computer bank which she was using to
analyse data developed a malfunction and over the next couple
of weeks similar breakdowns occurred whenever she used
computer equipment. On a few occasions an apparent corre-
spondence was noticed between her proximity to the computer
bank and sporadic changes in rotation speed of the tape reels.

> Usually the computers operated normally again after RA
> left the room. No one could explain the temporary break-
> downs but observers said they resembled a circuit
> overload. The incidence of this effect gradually dimin-
> ished but has not completely ceased. Recently [the report
> was published in 1979, some eighteen months after my
> visit] a similar difficulty developed with other equipment
> in the laboratory where RA conducts her research. She
> reports that these effects occur most often when she is
> upset. She does not claim to possess any unusual psychic
> ability but has stated that perhaps MM's guidance helped
> her 'exteriorize some innate capacities'. No effort is being
> made to follow up this possibility in any systematic way.
> RA is afraid that any publicity would interfere with her
> professional career.

I had more fun with the researchers in California than with any
previous group of scientists. Many of them were young and those
who were significantly older did not appear to hold my youth-

fulness against me. The atmosphere was friendly and relaxed and I enjoyed being in their company socially. Sometimes a topic of conversation would spark an informal experiment, such as when one of the researchers and I decided to find out what effect, if any, drugs had on telepathic ability. He smoked a joint of cannabis while I mentally transmitted symbols to him. The drug had about the same effect as alcohol – because it induces a relaxed state, it tends to improve telepathic ability.

We took the experiment a stage further the following evening, when the researcher substituted LSD for cannabis. Given that LSD is a hallucinogenic and produces images, this was bound to make him 'see' something, even if it was not what I was sending out. He received a lot of strong images, as expected, but about an hour after he had taken the drug, something very strange happened. I began to feel as though I had taken the drug too. I became extremely sensitive to everything around me and had a weird sensation of looking out of my head through two black holes. I was aware of my consciousness streaming out through my eye-sockets all over the floor and paddling around in it.

Rolling Thunder's words about not getting out of step within the medicine wheel came back to me afterwards. I had always regarded drugs and alcohol as potentially damaging to the individual who takes them. This experience made me appreciate how the damage can spill over and affect the lives of the people around that individual. It was a lesson I would later forget to my cost.

An interesting postscript to my experiences in California was added some years later when I talked to Uri Geller in depth for the first time. It was widely suggested at the time – and subsequently found to be true, according to Geller's biographer, Jonathan Margolis – that work he had done at the Stanford Research Institute in California was funded by the CIA. The US intelligence agencies had been following the lead of their Soviet counterparts who, it was believed, were spending millions of dollars on 'psychic warfare'.

All of the research done with me at Davis was allegedly unfunded and conducted in the spare time of the various researchers. This is probably true in so far as the University of California did not foot the bill. However, I am now fairly sure that a branch of the military, probably the US Navy, made those experiments possible.

An ESP test in which I participated was designed to gauge my ability to 'see' target drawings and was conducted in the presence of laser physicists Russell Targ and Hal Puthoff, under the aegis of the Nuclear Science Division of Lawrence Berkeley Laboratory. Targ and Puthoff had conducted a series of telepathy tests with Uri Geller in 1972 and 1974 and were involved in the secret remote-viewing programme at Fort Meade, Maryland, which was instigated and funded by the CIA. Under this programme dozens of intelligence agents with psychic ability were trained to psychically project themselves inside military installations such as submarines and nuclear missile silos.

At the time I looked on the physiological experiments conducted by Fred Lorenz as having purely medical applications, especially the test with the frog skin. In retrospect, a more sinister motive may explain the researchers' interest in whether I could influence somebody's brain-wave pattern or sympathetic nervous system at a distance and to what degree. Perhaps if I had been asked to stop the heart of a pig – as was a shocked Uri Geller – I would have been more suspicious sooner. Almost twenty years later it seems inconceivable that governments would involve themselves in this kind of research, but then fear that the Soviet Union might be stealing a march on the US militarily was reason enough.

An ironic aspect of those California experiments was the number of times the scientists were frustrated by inexplicable glitches. Lorenz and his researchers reported 'an unusual number of problems'. Two attempts to monitor my heartbeat using a heart-rate coupler failed when the coupler stopped working for no apparent reason. After the first failure the coupler functioned normally after I left the laboratory later in the day and behaved itself during the control tests the following morning. However, just before the second attempt, it malfunctioned again. The engineer who inspected it could find nothing wrong. The apparatus was subsequently returned to the manufacturer. Technicians there could find nothing wrong either and sent it back to Lorenz, who said that it had been functioning well since its return.

Lorenz reported 'disconcerting results' when he tried to specify random arouse/sedate sequences for tests on the sympathetic nervous system:

> At first we entered a table of random numbers, using odd numbers for arousal and even numbers for sedation, but each time we obtained abnormally long sequences of odd or even. Then I turned to tossing a coin and obtained nine heads in a row. I refused to use that and made two further attempts, both of which led to long sequences of the same face before being abandoned. I wish I had completed these and kept an accurate record. The probability must have been astronomical. At the time, however, I simply felt frustrated in trying to get an experiment started, and finally resorted to preparing cards with equal numbers of 'arouse' and 'sedate' orders, shuffling these and drawing them at random.
>
> The experimental results were also frequently frustrating. As I watched the pen writer during the experiments I felt that in most cases I could see the pen move in a consistent and significant manner in response to an order. However, there was so much 'noise' in the records that later attempts to interpret them were essentially fruitless. Only a few records were clear enough to analyze ...

Such frustrations apart, the scientists in California considered their time with me to have been largely well spent. In the report on the experiments ('A Month with Matthew Manning') published some months later, Jeffrey Mishlove wrote in the introduction: 'Taken as a whole, our month-long experience with Matthew

Manning has yielded sufficient evidence to refute the arguments of those who would maintain that Manning is a fraud.'

* * *

I left San Francisco on 17 June for the East Coast and the start of my public-speaking engagements for an educational organization called the Human Development Center. Between 19 June and the end of July they were running a series of conferences at colleges in Erie, Pennsylvania, North Easton, Massachusetts and Staten Island, New York. Entitled 'Your Psychic Self', each conference was devoted to exploring and developing psychic potential. I was one of the conference 'leaders' whose job it was to guide the participants' psychic development. The other 'leaders' included mediums, hypnotherapists, healers and psychics who were used to teaching and working with groups.

I felt very green because I had only my experiences to share with the people who came to hear me. I gave talks on the poltergeist, telekinesis and ESP, and led workshops on automatic writing and directing psychic energy. I had no trouble finding an audience, although I am not sure how many of those participants I helped to get in touch with their psychic selves. Although I was the new kid on the block, fortunately the conference participants – predominantly middle aged and female – saw something in what was being offered. My Englishness helped enormously. Americans seem to love the sound of English voices and the English capacity for understatement.

The people who attended these conferences were at the very least open minded about psychic phenomena. Some were open minded to the point of naivety, but it made a refreshing change not to have my word constantly challenged or to be regarded with suspicion. In the world beyond this safe haven the sceptics of psychic phenomena, led by the magicians, were still having a heyday attacking their arch-enemies, the psychics.

I had to get back for the launch of *In the Minds of Millions* on 15 August and be available for the inevitable round of interviews.

A special event was being organized with the *Sunday Mirror*, which was running extracts from the book, beginning with the 24 July issue and ending on the eve of the book's publication. Peter Bander had negotiated a good deal with the paper: £15,000 for the serialization rights. My stock had risen considerably since publication of *The Link*, for which the *Mail* had paid a mere £2,000.

The *Mirror* were keen to engage their readers beyond merely providing them with entertaining copy from the book, and sent out an invitation to help test my 'incredible powers'. Readers were asked to tune in to me telepathically between 6 p.m. and 6.15 p.m. on Sunday 7 August. At this time I would be at the top of London's Post Office Tower transmitting to them three mental images known only to me and the newspaper's editor.

This was an adaptation of an experiment I had conducted in Stockholm, where I had successfully sent thoughts telepathically while being flown low over a suburb of the city in a light aircraft. The aim of both experiments from my perspective was to show that psychic abilities are not confined to a select few and that many people possess them in varying degrees. My recent workshops in the States had been based on the same premise, that psychic ability is relevant to everyone and can be used in practical ways.

The *Mirror's* readers were told that between 6 and 6.05 p.m. I would be transmitting a colour; between 6.05 and 6.10 p.m. I would be concentrating my mind on a three-figure number, and between 6.10 and 6.15 I would be thinking about a shape or outline. I advised readers to try to clear their minds and to concentrate on me and the Post Office Tower for the full fifteen minutes. The newspaper asked people to write in with details of what they believed had been in my mind.

More than 25 per cent of the 2,500 postcards received by the newspaper gave at least one of the three images correctly. Nearly a quarter of readers who responded correctly gave the colour green. (I had found this the most difficult of the three to 'transmit' because there were red and blue decorations all around me in the Top of the Tower restaurant.) One in 50 gave the number 123 correctly, and around one in 30 received a shape that was identifiable as a house. Statistically, this was far beyond the bounds of coincidence, according to the expert the paper consulted, Michael Haslam, Deputy Honorary Secretary of the Institute of Statisticians: 'The probability of these results happening by chance are more than a thousand to one against. It's way off the end of my statistical scales,' he said.

Readers were warned that 'strange things could happen' in their homes when I concentrated my psychic energy. After the experiment, 'scores of reports' were received by the paper of personal items being affected by my transmission. 'Dozens said that their broken clocks, watches, radios, tape recorders, music boxes and even electric lights began working after 6.15 on Sunday night.' One waggish reader wrote: 'As advised I placed a broken-down object in front of the TV set – my brother, who hasn't worked for years. He sat there open-mouthed. He is now working again.'

One publication had chronicled my career more thoroughly than any other – *Psychic News*, the house journal of the Spiritualist movement. In 1977 its editor was still Maurice Barbanell, who had founded the paper in 1932. Around the time of the publication of *In the Minds of Millions* he invited me to lunch at the Connaught to discuss my recent experiences in the States and my future plans.

Our conversation was interrupted when a heavy silver plate on an adjoining table rose up, turned over and crashed to the floor, causing consternation all around. Barbanell asked our waiter what had happened because so far as he could see nothing in the vicinity could have made it behave that unusually. The waiter shrugged and said, 'I don't think we've got a polter-geist here.' I was used to such happenings, and Barbanell had spent years reporting them. We both laughed.

In October I returned to the States to fulfil a series of speaking engagements and to take part in experiments with William Braud. He was an experimental psychologist and a former professor of psychology at the University of Houston who worked out of the Mind Science Foundation in San Antonio, Texas, which had been endowed in 1976 by the estate of Tom Slick, a San Antonio oilman.

Braud and his fellow researchers – Gary Davis and Robert Wood – were embarked upon a series of experiments involving psychokinetic influences upon biological systems, and it was these I was most interested in helping them with. However, these experiments were scheduled for January. The two experiments in which I was to participate on this trip involved clairvoyance. Neither experiment interested me and neither produced a startling result. The main value of the week was that it enabled Braud and his team to get to know me – and me them – before the important work ahead.

After Texas I flew to Toronto to visit George and Iris Owen, whom I had not seen since the New Horizons Conference in 1974. They were thoughtful hosts and made my short stay very pleasant.

One evening we were joined by a Detroit doctor, William Wolfson, and his wife Tracy and our conversation turned to Ted Serios. In the 1960s Serios had captured the attention of the public with his claim that he could produce what he called Thoughtographs by staring into the lens of a loaded Polaroid camera and concentrating, causing an image to appear on the unexposed film. He had experimented with different sorts of film and had found Polaroid to be the most easily influenced, probably because of its chemical make-up. Many of the images produced by Serios show clouds of light, and in some of them groups of figures and landscapes are discernible.

I had been more impressed by the results achieved by a Japanese boy who was working in a similar way to Serios. However, to manage to project anything at all onto film seemed startling and I wondered aloud how difficult it would be. No sooner had I spoken the words than the means arrived: George left the room and came back with a Polaroid camera and several rolls of unexposed film. He loaded the camera, which he then handed to Tracy, and asked me to pose as I would normally for a photograph and not to attempt to influence the camera.

The picture that came out is unremarkable and shows me sitting on a sofa looking relaxed. For the next shot he asked me to project energy towards the camera. I started to meditate on the idea of energy flowing through me, and when I could feel tingling in my hands I asked Tracy to take another photograph. In this image it looks as though mist is swirling around the room. By the time a third photograph was taken a few moments later the sensation in my hands had intensified and I could feel heat in them. In this image I can hardly be seen behind strong, white concentric rings of light, which remind me of the tunnel of light phenomenon given in many descriptions of near-death experience.

The film ran out at this point and a second roll was quickly inserted. In the next shot the concentric circles are even more pronounced, and neither I nor the room can be seen. George suggested that we try using a second camera and yet another roll of film to reduce the possibility of there being a fault with either the first camera or the first two rolls of film. I was beginning to feel tired and in need of a rest so we called a halt before trying a more ambitious idea.

When I was ready to continue, George asked me to create an energy field. Again, I started by meditating, emptying my mind of extraneous thoughts. Then I tried to imagine a large ball of light coming out of my head. The photograph taken by Tracy shows just such a ball, surrounded by faint circles of light. As we were looking at this image, George suggested that I try to transfer the energy to Iris. I knelt beside her as she sat on a chair and took her hand. The photograph taken of us together shows exactly the same ball coming out of her head.

A total of about seventy photographs must have been taken during that session in Toronto, and the vast majority of them reveal nothing exceptional. However, the images displaying the concentric rings of light and the energy ball came out in sequence and clearly show a development. I am still amazed by them, because they are so unlike other images I have seen.

People have sometimes pointed out faint spots of light evident in other photographs of me and taken these as signs of paranormal interference, but I am convinced that the Polaroids taken at the Owens' house are the only images of me that could be said to bear such an imprint.

After a few days I said goodbye to George and Iris and embarked on six weeks of talks and demonstrations across the Mid-West, taking in Wisconsin, Minnesota and Illinois. It was the first of the thirty-three tours in America I would undertake between 1977 and 1981 and the start of a new education. I felt that if I could succeed in America, I could succeed anywhere. At this time my only claim to fame in the States was *The Link* and if I wanted to be regarded for anything else I would have to prove myself. I had to start virtually from scratch and, ironically, learn to respect what I had previously tended to look down my nose at.

Those first 'conferences' earlier in the year had made me appreciate the value of entertainment in any public appearance. This was not high on the agenda of many of my fellow speakers and 'leaders', who tended to preach. The way to entertain, I decided, was to make the presentation as good as the content so that people would want to come and hear what I had to say.

My most vivid recollection of that autumn tour was an evening in Chicago. This consisted of a talk about my experiences followed by a demonstration of automatic writing. For the demonstration I would ask people in the audience to give me a name and then see if any information would come through me. That night I received a message whose content seemed odd and made no sense to me. I only realized this as I was reading it back to the person who had given me the name; I was oblivious of what was being written when I received these automatic communications. The person was clearly made very anxious by this information and tried to take away the piece of paper on which it was written. I often used to let people have these scraps of paper, but on this particular occasion something prompted me to keep it.

Shortly afterwards I received the first of several threatening telephone calls. The person at the other end of the line told me that if I wanted to remain in good health I should not on any account broadcast the information contained in the automatic message, or words to this effect. I was too taken aback to respond. This must be a common reaction because when the second threatening call came it was almost as though the man was making sure I had fully understood the content of his first call. There was no mistake. The threat was meant for me, and I should heed it.

I had every intention of taking the man at his word and told him so. The last thing I wanted was to come across as the sort of person who relishes the idea of a death-defying challenge. However, I reasoned that curiosity in the safety of my hotel room would not be harmful. I read the automatic message more carefully and eventually came to the conclusion that it concerned the assassination of President Kennedy and also a connection between the Mafia and US politicians. But its full significance remained unclear. I was glad to be leaving for home.

When I got back I destroyed the message and then did my best to persuade the people who felt threatened that it would impossible for me to re-establish contact with the original inform- ant. The tag 'psychic', which was routinely applied to me wherever I went, did not help and I had never liked it. I did not want to be thought of as having mediumistic abilities and it was this impres- sion that had surely panicked those people into threatening me.

I issued a statement through Peter Bander in which I made it clear that, in future, I wanted to be known as a mentalist, not a psychic. I kept to myself another decision I had made – to drop automatic writing from future public demonstrations. Until Chicago it had not occurred to me that people might be trying to use me for their own purposes. Now that I was aware of this possibility, I could not ignore it.

I do not know if calling myself a mentalist helped me get off the hook that had been put out for me in Chicago – certainly I received no more threats.

This was all still buzzing around in my head when I appeared on the *Russell Harty Show*, which was a very popular television chat show in the late 1970s. Like David Frost had done three years previously, Harty devoted the programme to me. Viewers could be forgiven for thinking that his production team had taken most of their ideas from the earlier programme. The events of *The Link* were rerun, and a clip of me doing automatic drawing was shown. The major difference came at the end of the show, when I attempted a couple of a telepathy experiments instead of doing Thomas Penn diagnoses.

The tour in the States had taught me how often things could go wrong and I was learning not to be embarrassed when, as on Harty's show, they did. A trick can be perfected. What I was doing could not. Psychokinetic energy cannot be turned on and off at will and made to produce results on cue every time. Failure worried me greatly to begin with because I regarded it as a negative measure of my ability, while success proved that I was not a fraud – which some people were trying to make me out to be.

If the Harty show did nothing else it prompted the satirical magazine *Private Eye* to immortalize me in its pages. A couple of months after that appearance, I discovered that I had made it into 'Great Bores of Today', a regular column reserved for people who were always in the media saying the same thing.

* * *

In mid January I left the English winter behind me and flew to Texas to complete the series of experiments with William Braud. Most of the experiments were designed to test what effect, if any, my thoughts would have on a range of biological systems. The first of the living systems was a gerbil. In the 'influence' trials I had to try to mentally urge the animal to become more active on an 'activity wheel'. During the trials I would sit and think about the gerbil in its natural habitat, which is the desert. I would imagine a hawk swooping down, talons outstretched for the kill, and the hapless animal running for its life. In the control runs, I was asked not to try to use this influence, so I would switch my attention away from the animal by reading a newspaper or magazine.

The clicking of the event marker of the polygraph record in the room where I was sitting gave me a rough idea of how the gerbil was reacting. What I could hear puzzled me, because it was exactly the reverse of what I was expecting. The polygraph indicated that whenever I used the image of the hawk the tread-mill slowed down and then stopped. As soon as I removed my attention from the gerbil, activity on the treadmill increased. Only later did we discover that when a gerbil feels threatened by a predator it will instinctively freeze on the spot and not, as I had envisaged, run for its life.

Braud then asked me to use my mind on a more familiar animal. Ten volunteer humans were hooked up to a lie detector, which was adjusted to record sweat-gland activity in their hands. I was in a distant room where I could not see the volunteers but could see the lie detector readings.

A pack of twenty shuffled cards was placed in front of me. Half of the cards bore an instruction to do nothing, the other half an instruction to attempt to increase the level of tension in the volunteers. When I was instructed to do the latter I would imagine some emotional situation that might confront the person – for example, seeing an accident or coming across a scary object. Braud told the *National Enquirer*'s reporter, Charles Parminter, 'After the experiment the volunteers told me they felt the influence Matthew was having on them. They felt more tense. In some cases they actually felt as though he was in the room shaking them.'

The lie detector recorded that the anxiety levels in these people had risen by an average of 9 per cent, a result that Braud described as 'quite impressive'.

The experiment that most interested me involved my trying to heal red blood cells (erythrocytes). I was asked to use psycho-kinesis to influence the rate of haemolysis, or abnormal degeneration, of these cells. If red blood cells are put in ordinary tap water the red corpuscles will expand and eventually burst, releasing haemoglobin. However, if that water is made slightly saline the red corpuscles are buffered and they keep intact longer. As haemolysis proceeds the appearance of the blood-saline solution changes from cloudy to clear, allowing more and more light to pass through them and providing researchers with a measure of the rate of decay.

The experiment consisted of ten runs, scheduled on ten successive days. Each run involved rate of haemolysis measures on ten blood samples. Five of these were control samples and five were samples that I attempted to influence. For the control runs I attempted not to think of the tube. When I was trying to influence I put my hands above but not touching the tube and imagined the cells surrounded with brilliant white light. I assured the cells that the light and energy would protect them and that they would remain intact and resistant to the solution.

Braud's results showed that the cells lasted intact four times longer in the experiments in which I tried to 'heal' than they did in the experiments where my influence was absent. In an interview with the *National Enquirer*, Braud said: 'By concentrating his mind on the test tube of blood, Matthew was able to slow down the death of cells. Normally the blood cells would break down and die within a maximum of five minutes. But he was able to slow down the destruction so that the blood cells were still intact as long as twenty minutes later.'

In one of these experiments the protocol was changed so that instead of sitting next to Braud with my hands above the test tubes, I sat in a room thirty metres away and attempted to influence their contents at a distance. Braud had no idea whether I was trying to influence the blood in the test tubes or not. Instructions were given to me separately via a deck of cards, indicating which mode I should adopt. Interestingly, the result of this experiment departed even more from chance expectation.

Unusually among scientists, Braud had a genuine interest in assessing the potential of psychic healing and it was thanks to him that I undertook a series of experiments that would set me on the path to direct healing. He arranged for me to do trials with Dr John Kmetz of the Science Unlimited Research Foundation, which was also based in San Antonio. The purpose of these experiments was to see if I could disrupt the charge on Hela cervical cancer cells to render them inactive.

Named after Henrietta Lafayette, the black American woman from whom they were taken before her death in the 1950s, these cells are used extensively in cancer research laboratories around the world. The cells are grown in culture flasks (plastic containers that look similar to the cases of audio cassette tapes) in a liquid protein feed. When the cells are first put in the flask they float in the liquid. Eventually they will drop to the bottom of the flask, where they begin to grow.

After a period of several days the cells will cover the bottom surface of the flask, attaching themselves to the plastic by means of an electrostatic force produced by the positive/negative attraction between the cells and the flask – the cells themselves have a positive charge on their surface, while the flask has a negative charge. Kmetz had been working with two healers who in experiments had disrupted the charge on the surface of the cell, causing the cell to float free in the medium in which it had been grown. In this state the cell is essentially inactive or dead.

Some amount of cell death normally occurs in the tissue culture (usually in the order of about 1,000 cells per millilitre of liquid), so before each trial the researchers used a machine called a spectrophotometer to count the number of dead cancer cells to give them a control line or measure of the 'state of health' of the cultures. Each culture flask was sealed with wax – to ensure that any attempt to physically break open the flask would be obvious – and then placed on a level surface for me to influence.

It was my job for the next twenty minutes to try to give healing to the cells. In some of the thirty trials I was allowed to hold the flask between my hands, and in others I attempted to influence the cultures at a distance, while confined in an electrically shielded room. Somebody else who was not a healer was also given a flask of cells and had the job of mimicking every movement I made. A third container was left in another part of the building and received no attention.

I tried to envisage the cells surrounded by white light and imagined I was talking to them. I told them that their purpose on this level of reality was ended and they had to go elsewhere. After each experiment Dr Kmetz put the samples back in the spectrophotometer and re-counted them.

In each of the thirty trials there was never any change in the number of dead cells in the container that had been left in a different part of the building. Neither was there any change in the number of dead cells in the container that the other person tried to influence in imitation of me. However, in 27 out of the 30 trials there was a change in the number of cells in the flask I tried to influence, ranging in magnitude from 200 to 1,200 per cent changes. If at the beginning of the trial there was 1 dead cell per millilitre of liquid, after my intervention there were anything from 2 to 12 dead cells.

Braud, who observed these trials first-hand, described the results as 'impressive' and concluded: 'What Matthew has demonstrated is that he can influence cancer cells. There may be parapsychological factors involved that could be used to heal oneself or heal others.' In a television interview Kmetz talked about the experiment's significance:

> If we can translate this now to an individual who has a tumour, what we would like to have these individuals who are acting as healers do is to affect the tumour perhaps in the same way as they are affecting the cells in the culture, and cause the cell metabolism to decrease to the point where you get dissolution of the tumour, and have the tumour breaking up.

I was greatly encouraged by what these two respected scientists had to say about the experiment. It was a revelation, a validation.

I had wanted to discover practical applications for the gift I had been given. It seemed there was nothing to stop me turning my attention from the contents of test tubes to human beings and having the same positive effect.

The experiments with Braud and Kmetz were essential in instilling in me a necessary but hitherto missing ingredient: self-belief. Until this point I had not believed I could heal directly – this gift I allowed only to 'giants' like Harry Edwards and Rolling Thunder – and whether I could or could not heal did not seem relevant. My role was to offer myself as a guinea pig to help competent, committed scientists explore the possibilities of healing energy. Now I knew what those possibilities were.

* * *

Anita Gregory, the principal researcher of the Society for Psychical Research (SPR), had readily agreed to my suggestion that we do experiments together. Soon after I returned from the States, we met to discuss what form the experiments should take. I told her that I was keen to try to replicate some of the biological tests I had done in the States with William Braud.

It quickly became apparent that Anita Gregory's major interest was in attempting to replicate some ground-breaking experiments conducted in the 1930s with Rudi Schneider, who she looked upon as the definitive twentieth-century physical medium. He had taken part in experiments with Eugène Osty, Director of the Institut Métaphysique in Paris, and his son Marcel, an engineer, who devised a sort of infra-red burglar-alarm system to guard objects which Schneider was attempting to move by psychic means. In experiments with Osty and subsequently with other researchers, the alarm was repeatedly triggered whenever Schneider, speaking as his control personality 'Olga', announced that he would move such and such an object. In Osty's view, Schneider, when in a trance, exteriorized some force which was invisible in white light but detectable by means of infra-red radiation of suitable wavelength.

Infra-red equipment which Anita Gregory had had specially designed to test the same phenomenon was ready and waiting for a suitable subject to come along and offer his services. I was not offering, because I was no longer interested in trying to influence machines. However, I was prepared to be persuaded if more interesting experiments could also be arranged. Consequently, she invited several other researchers to design some biological tests.

All the experiments were to be financed by the Koestler Foundation, which had been set up by Arthur Koestler, Dr Brian Inglis and the financier Instone ('Tony') Bloomfield. Anita Gregory suggested that I bring a friend on experiment days, to keep me company and to act as my witness. Out of the several names I put forward, she chose Brian Inglis. I had first met Brian at the press conference given by Corgi when *The Link* came out in paperback. From that point on he had supported me publicly, sometimes through his column in the *Evening Standard*, and we had become friends.

Brian's views and enthusiasms were essentially anti-establishment, and he was conventional only in his appearance and manner of speaking. He was the most unjournalist-like journalist I have met, being entirely free of spite or ambition. His charm and basic decency attracted many people to him, especially women. None of these admirers, however, managed to change his Bohemian bachelor ways. Being used to the ultra-tidiness of my home in Linton, I was shocked the first time I entered his basement flat in Belsize Park. Papers and books covered virtually every surface, including the floor space, which had to be carefully negotiated via narrow pathways between the piles. I have never seen a place like it. Even Brian's taste in alcohol was unique. His favourite brew was a mix of Guinness and champagne.

All of the SPR experiments, biological or otherwise, turned out to be a real grind for me. Perhaps I had been spoiled by my recent experiences in the States, but I expected to be treated as an equal and to feel a rapport with the researchers. The worst aspect was that most of them did not seem particularly interested in proving anything. If the report of the experiments is an accurate guide to intent, nor did they seem to expect to: '. . . [T]he two weeks were regarded as a period of concentrated exploration, rather than providing definitive results'. I found this attitude very irksome.

The 'lightning flashes and dramatic psi' which, Braud noted, I had exhibited throughout my visit to Texas were singularly lacking in London. The reasons for this were plain enough. I got the distinct impression that the experiments I wanted to do were merely making up the numbers, supporting acts to Anita Gregory's homage to Rudi Schneider. This did not help my motivation which, as William Braud had demonstrated statistically in his report on our experiments together, was extremely important if I was to give of my best.

The infra-red equipment was set up all the time in a laboratory at London's City University where the experiments were conducted, dominating the proceedings psychologically. I regarded it as an enemy. The experimentation area was organized so that attention could be switched from project to project, thus achieving maximum flexibility. That was the theory. The reality was that I felt like someone who is being pressurized to cook several uninteresting meals at once.

My success in influencing the infra-red beam began almost spontaneously, without any real concentration or effort from me. I was feeling very irritated and bored because a haemolysis experiment I was expecting to do was delayed while the experimenter, Professor William Byers Brown, made adjustments to his equipment. Anita Gregory thought this would be a good time for me to try the first poetry experiment; in this I had to draw a picture that was unambiguously relevant to or illustrative of a poem that was concealed in a package.

This was similar to one of the 'incidental' experiments involving clairvoyance I had taken part in with William Braud in Texas. In this I had been asked to draw the content of a 35-mm slide sealed inside an opaque envelope. In his report, Braud had described the result as 'quite impressive'. I sketched a picture containing two palm trees, three birds, a castle, a horizon, a sun, converging lines terminating in a gate or door, and an anchor on its side, with one of its points resting on a cracked egg. The hidden slide had actually contained two palm trees, one bird, an architectural structure resembling the top of a castle, an ocean horizon, an apple held between two fingers in such a way that it resembled the two points of the anchor and the egg, a bush and two people.

Anita and I agreed that the first drawing I completed in the SPR experiment was reasonably relevant. I could see no correspondences in any of the three further drawings I produced. Nor could Anita Gregory. One of the other researchers, however, Mary Rose Barrington, persisted in trying to find them, and sometimes went to ludicrous lengths trying to explain the relationships between my drawings and lines in the poems. No doubt she was motivated by kindness, and was trying to encourage me, but all she succeeded in doing was exasperating me and everyone else present.

I got up and started stalking around the infra-red equipment. How easy would it be, I wondered, to influence the equipment? But this thought was quickly overcome by another, which told me that there was no point in bothering because no one was there to take any interest. Anita Gregory had left the room, and Professor Arthur Ellison was not there either. Only Mary Rose Barrington and David Chapman, a research assistant in Ellison's Department of Electrical and Electronic Engineering at City University, were in the room.

I started smacking my right fist into the palm of my left hand, a characteristic gesture I still make when I feel frustrated. Soon severe irregularities manifested in the printout. Several times that afternoon and on subsequent days similar bouts of deflection were recorded. One day the read-out showed an irregularity that came to be known as the 'Grattan-Guinness peak'. It came about as follows.

Dr Ivor Grattan-Guinness had initially expressed interest in being part of the SPR's investigating team but lost it when he discovered that the experiments would clash with his holiday. Whether he was bored or did not want to miss out on being associated with the experiments, I do not know, but he rang Anita Gregory from where he was holidaying in Devon and told her that he and his wife, Enid, intended to 'send' some telepathic messages starting the following day precisely at noon.

When Anita related their intention to me the next morning, I told her that if they could not be bothered to be present in person, I could not be bothered to accommodate their inane plan. More importantly, the haemolysis experiment with Professor William Byers Brown scheduled for that morning held far more promise. However, shortly before noon and for about fifteen minutes after this deadline, I found my attention switching from the blood cells to the infra-red machine. During this period the chart trace left the baseline and made a shape never previously nor subsequently observed.

During some of the sessions I would clench my fists and tense my muscles before jumping up and down, making wide circular movements with my arms. By the end of the first week my muscles were so strained from this activity that I could barely scratch my back. I had no particular conscious thoughts when I was trying to influence the machine, only a great determination that I should be successful. According to the report on the experiments, Professor Ellison and Roger Chapman, Senior Lecturer in Engineering and a member of Ellison's staff, expressed the view that 'he had not seen apparatus behaving like this before and can find no normal engineering explanation'.

An experiment involving a machine that generates numbers at random, also conducted by Ellison, caused similar perplexity. This was basically a clairvoyance test to 'see' random numbers. The American psychic Ingo Swann had recently performed trials with this same equipment and caused it to behave oddly. The competitive urge to see if I could have the same effect as Swann was strong enough to make me agree to try the experiment, even though I felt it was a waste of time. I knew I could make the generator go wrong. When I concentrated on Ellison's machine, it repeatedly produced the number 8, as it had for Ingo Swann, indicating a fault in the microcircuits. No obvious fault in these could be found, and subsequently the machine returned to normal functioning.

The haemolysis experiment devised by Professor Brown was a big disappointment for me personally. Twice we attempted to replicate the results achieved in Texas but without success. Brown and I did not succeed either in replicating the rapport that had existed between myself and William Braud. This, I am sure, was the principal reason for the experiment's failure. Braud had been supportive and pleasant to have around, and because of his personal attributes there had been a great atmosphere in the laboratory. Brown was like some nineteenth-century schoolmaster in comparison. He was as aware of the mismatch as I was and kept fussing about having a 'negative experimenter effect' on me.

Repeated carefully controlled experiments suggest strongly that some experimenters are much more likely to achieve positive results with given subjects than are other experimenters. In a talk to the California Society for Psychical Research, given in October 1977, Fred Lorenz described what he calls 'Murphy's Law', defined as 'If anything can possibly go wrong, it will, and at the worst possible time':

> I've been very much intrigued for many years with the possible effect of people on people ... and why some experiments go and some don't ... There are some people who seem to be able to turn out successful experiments one after the other and erect tremendous bibliographies and develop a fantastic amount of material. And others struggle along, and keep making mistakes, and things just go wrong for no good reason ... I've sometimes suspected that the experimenter has effects on the subjects, and vice versa, that are unexpected and unexplained.

Other commitments kept Brian Inglis from attending on most days. When he was not there his place was taken by Ruth West, who ran the Koestler Foundation. The two of them ended up acting as a sort of buffer between me and the Society's scientists. Ruth was also interested to see how the Foundation's money was being spent, as was Tony Bloomfield, the Koestler Foundation's main financial backer, who visited the laboratory one day.

Although Brian did not have much faith in the SPR's scientists, he was hoping that the results of the experiments would be worth reporting to the wider world. One of the newspaper contacts he brought along one day to observe the experiments in progress was Bill (later Lord) Deedes, then the editor of the *Daily Telegraph*, who expressed interest in carrying a story on the results when they were published. Not surprisingly, his interest waned during the four years it took the SPR to publish their report.

Mary Rose Barrington's mung bean experiment sums up my feelings about the time I spent at the SPR's disposal. The first experiment produced promising results: of the 48 beans in which I tried to encourage growth, 42 displayed radicles after seven days of growth; this compared with 32 in the control group.

While trying to influence the beans I imagined that I was expanding my consciousness as far as I could – out through the walls, across London and beyond, into space – until I was as one with the space and energy was coming through me, filling my hands. At this point I put my hands over the seeds and imagined them in an atmosphere where they had everything they needed to sprout very quickly.

I repeated this exercise with a second tray of beans, which were then put into the care of a biology teacher, the aptly named Mr Fudge, for cultivation. Unfortunately, he did not get around to attending to them until four weeks later, because, according to Miss Barrington's report, 'the persons concerned were living at some distance from one another and had other commitments'. Not surprisingly, the encouraging result with the first lot of beans was not replicated.

I wonder if that second tray of beans was the one Miss Barrington took home with her and placed on a sideboard in her sitting room. A tray of what she called 'treated' beans was in residence when one evening she, her mother and a visiting friend were discussing psychical matters and heard a loud explosive report coming from the direction of the sideboard. The three of them immediately supposed that the light bulb in the lamp on the sideboard had 'blown'. However, neither this nor any other bulb, or the television tube, was found to be damaged.

Miss Barrington, a solicitor in her professional life, was the subject of another strange occurrence during the period of the experiments. One Saturday evening when I was giving a lecture, she and Anita Gregory were at her home preparing some paper-work for the experiments when they heard 'four or five exceedingly loud but dull thuds', which 'sounded as if a muffled battering ram were hammering against the walls of the house immediately adjacent to where [they] were sitting'.

Miss Barrington 'immediately investigated all conceivable possible normal sources of these noises'. She subsequently ascer-tained that at the precise time this hammering was heard, a client of hers was badly wanting to speak to her about her case but dared not ring out of office hours. Many years previously this client had on several occasions reported hearing loud hammer-ing noises coming from her ceiling.

The report of the experiments I did with the SPR did not appear until four years later and was included in the Proceedings for October 1982, which marked the Society's centenary year. The report is disappointingly inconclusive, despite the results being mainly positive. It seemed to me that they had used the time to dismantle the material to such an extent that they could not answer their own questions. Unfortunately, too few of the Society's members are scientists and their ability to design exper-iments that further understanding of paranormal phenomena seems very limited.

However, at the end of 4 August 1978, the last day of the series of SPR experiments, I was feeling more charitable, and confident that what had happened justified the word 'success-ful' being applied to the experiments. Given the numerous tests in which I had taken part, I had surely done enough to silence my critics and prove something into the bargain. But I knew it was time to draw a line and step away. I had gone about as far as was possible in the laboratory. After India I had wondered how it would be possible for me to heal. Piece by piece the answers had been given to me, first in California, most recently in Texas. My future had been quietly taking shape, waiting for me to have the courage to step into it. I needed to work with people who would be prepared to trust my ability as much as I did.

Chapter 4

TREADING THE
BOARDS

The right time always makes itself known to us and cannot be ignored. I was at home in Linton one afternoon when a stranger came to the front door and introduced himself. He was an Italian doctor. I do not recall his name. He explained that his mother was seriously ill with cancer and was presently in Addenbrookes Hospital, Cambridge, which specialized in the liver transplant procedure that he had hoped might save her life and had prompted him to bring her to England. The specialists at the hospital, however, had declined to operate because she was so ill. In desperation he had come to me, having heard about the cancer-cell experiment I had done with John Kmetz in Texas. Would I, he asked, be prepared to go and treat his mother in hospital? I hesitated. I had not given healing before and although I knew I should be able to do it, I was momentarily daunted. My doubts were eventually no match for his pleading. I could not refuse to help and together we left for the hospital.

I remember receiving a terrible shock when I met his mother for the first time. Liver failure had caused her eyes and skin to yellow with jaundice. She was very emaciated, felt dizzy, was vomiting constantly and had a fever. I let my intuition guide me and did what I felt was right, very gently placing my hands on her and entering the mode I had adopted for the cancer-cell experiments. My intuition also told me when to stop, and after about fifteen minutes I took my leave, having agreed to return during visiting hours that evening.

When I went back I found the woman sitting in an armchair

in the corner of the room. Her temperature had returned to normal, the nausea and the pain had disappeared, and she had recovered her appetite. I was told she had eaten a meal and, to the amazement of the nurses, had kept it down, which she had not been able to do for weeks. I was very gratified by these signs of improvement and knew then that healing worked on people in the same way that it worked in test tubes. It was arranged that I should visit her again at lunchtime on the following day.

My feelings of self-congratulation were short-lived, however. The next morning I received a phone call from the woman's son, who told me that his mother had died during the night. His kind words of thanks could not lessen the sense of failure I experienced as the news of her death sank in. I had been so sure of being able to save her that the significance of the manner of her dying escaped me at the time.

What appeared to be a setback would gradually reveal its true nature as a blessing in disguise. Ego has no place in healing and on that first occasion I had been in danger of letting it intrude, merely by being so confident of 'success'. Healing is about more than miracle cures. In the case of that woman it helped her to meet death peacefully, free of fear, without pain and in dignity.

However, at this point my definition of success was not as rounded as it would subsequently become and my confidence in my ability to heal was shaken for months afterwards. I reasoned that inexperience lay at the root of my failure and gradually began to introduce healing demonstrations into my work. The positive results from these encouraged me to continue.

The States had at that time the most highly developed 'alternative' scene of any country in the world. The opportunities on offer there enabled me to marry my ambitions to be a healer with the necessity of earning a living. America is synonymous with competition and the American attitude of only the best being good enough produces a lot of people who are brilliant at what they do. The US suited my wide streak of perfectionism and encouraged me to take risks.

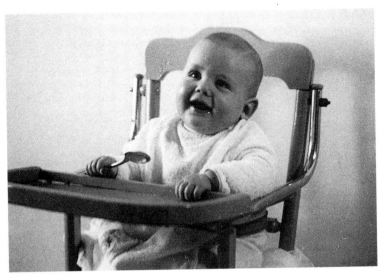

My earliest failed attempt at metal bending, aged nine months.

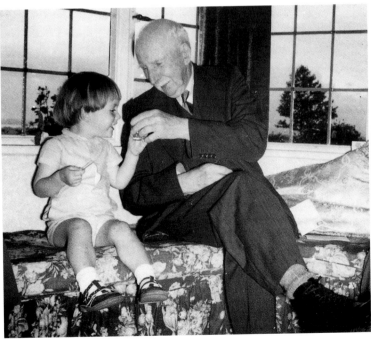

Sharing a discovery with my great-grandfather, who started out in life with minimal prospects and ended up owning a string of racehorses.

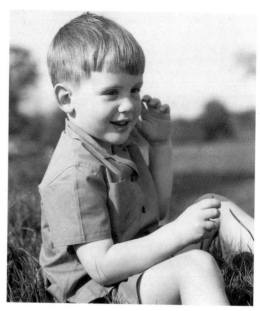

Aged four, during a visit to Whipsnade Zoo in Buckinghamshire. I may look compliant but my mother remembers this trip for my display of awkwardness and obstinacy.

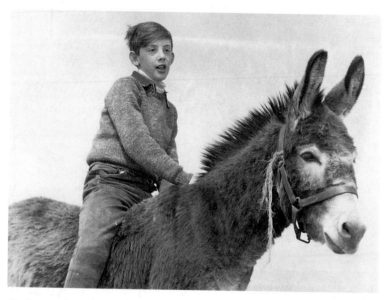

Getting away from it all. This photograph was taken during the Easter holidays of 1967, just after the first poltergeist incident at home.

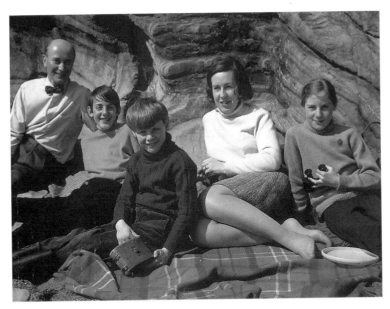

The whole family on holiday in the Scilly Isles later in 1967. By this time the poltergeist activity had subsided and we thought we had experienced the last of it. My brother Andrew is in the centre foreground, my sister Rosalind is at far right.

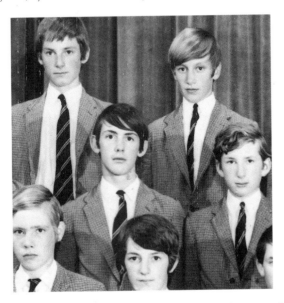

The poltergeist activity started up again in our new home at Linton in the summer of 1970 and in early 1971 – the year of this photograph – followed me to Oakham School. I am in the centre.

I died in Switzerland on
April 21 1952. I am now
restless. My body is at Sapperton
Where is Faith Hill? In the
Storm and uncertainty and fear
that today permeate the world,
set yourselves to become part of
the hand of God which stretches
out to bring peace and patience
and high standards of truth
and justice to all peoples. Bless
my body and allow mass. Here is
Charles, father now. I must go

Stafford Cripps

52.
T.

An example of automatic writing, purporting to come from statesman Sir Stafford Cripps.
After examining this in detail, the graphologist Vernon Harrison stated that if the signature
were appended to a will he would have to pass it for probate as genuine.

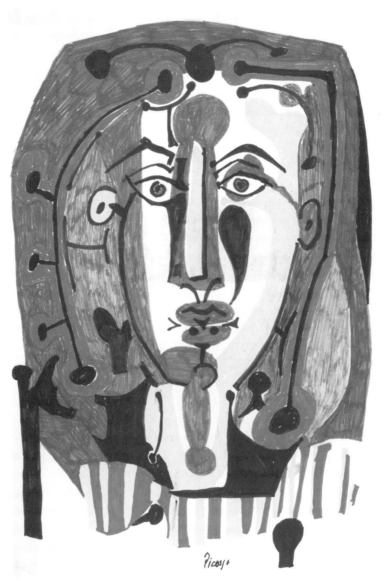

My mother suggested that I should try automatic drawing by attempting to contact a well-known artist and asking him to draw something for me. This example is in the style of Picasso. (Colin Smythe Ltd.)

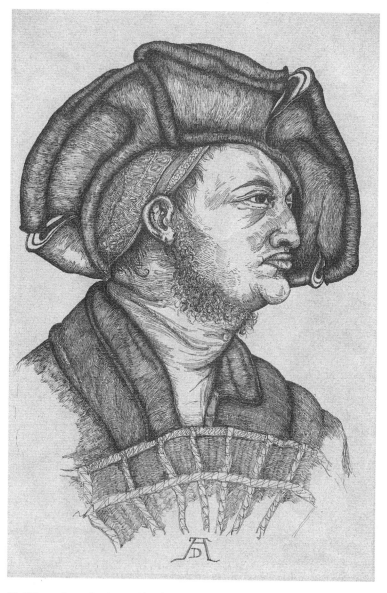

My Dürer-style pen drawing was identified as a version of a portrait of Ulrich Varnbüler, the preparatory drawing for which is held in the Albertina, Vienna. A print from the woodcut derived from the drawing in the Albertina is to be found in the Department of Prints and Drawings at the British Museum.   (Mr and Mrs D. Manning)

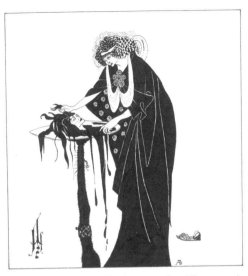

I was not considered to have any artistic talent by my teachers. The automatic drawings that came through me were in a variety of styles and often, like this drawing in the style of Aubrey Beardsley, were executed during lessons.

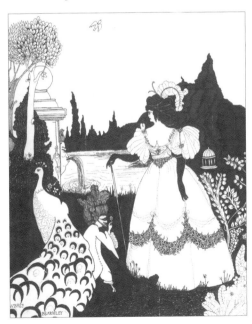

Vernon Harrison discovered that this picture was a composite of two Beardsley forgeries that were published around 1919 in a privately printed book. Many poor details in the forgeries seem to have been 'corrected' in my version.   (Colin Smythe Ltd.)

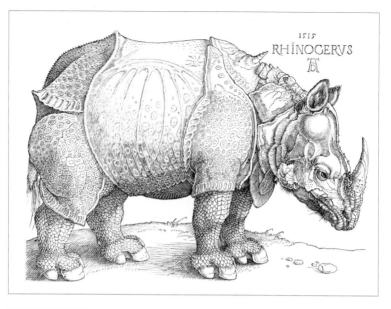

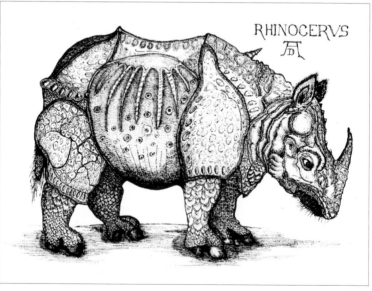

The top illustration is an original Dürer currently housed in the British Museum in London. (British Museum)

The lower illustration is a drawing which came through me.   (Colin Smythe Ltd.)

I would not perhaps have taken quite such an unusual route if I had not made the acquaintance of a remarkable young man at one of the 'alternative' conferences where we were both appearing. He was an ordinary guy with no psychic ability who had developed an extrordinary degree of control over his body. He could, for example, switch his pulse off on one side of his body, start it again and then repeat the exercise on the other side. No trickery was involved in this, as he proved by stripping down to his boxer shorts, putting both arms out and having people check his pulse.

We got on very well and talked about our plans for the future. I told him about my ambition to bring healing to a wider public than the committed alternative-lifestylers who seemed to make up the audiences attending my demonstrations. My new friend suggested that I might consider appearing on the night-club circuit, which was earning him a very good living. When I witnessed the rest of his repertoire, I understood how this could be.

In one demonstration he would lay a large tarpaulin on the ground and throw quantities of broken glass onto it. He would invite members of the audience to smash bottles and add these fragments to the debris, encouraging them to set up as many jagged edges as they liked. Wearing only boxer shorts, he would lie down on this bed of broken glass and then have men stand on his legs and chest. I saw him suffer cuts only afterwards, when he was clearing up the debris.

His demonstration with a wolf trap was perhaps even more incredible. He would start by showing what damage the trap could do, setting the trap, placing a twelve-inch wooden ruler in its open jaws, and then springing the trap, shearing the ruler in half. A member of the audience would set the trap again. This time he would put his hand where the ruler had been, springing the trap. Somehow he did not injure himself.

Night-club owners in the States were prepared to give anyone a chance to help them increase their takings, and I was no exception. My new friend arranged the necessary introductions and we began working together in these off-beat venues. We would work any place that was prepared to take us. The money was good, but I earned every cent. Getting the attention of people who are not interested in you or what you are doing is not easy, and keeping it can be even harder. Up to this point I had been able to rely on being known and admired by a hard core of devotees. Those people created a supportive atmosphere.

In the night-clubs I faced clusters of bodies who were there principally to eat, drink and have a good time with their friends. I was an extra they could take or leave, as their mood dictated. It was a salutary experience, and the best of all training grounds. Shy though I was, I relished the challenge of finding a way of reaching this new audience. It represented a genuine cross-section of ordinary people, and I could not rely on a shared background, age or interests to see me through.

I was hoping that the report by John Kmetz would lead to healing making a bigger impact on public consciousness. During a visit to the States in April 1978 I had telephoned Kmetz to enquire how his report was progressing. He had enthused over the results and said he was keen to see them replicated elsewhere. When a full year after the experiments I had still not received a formal report, I decided to press harder.

By this time I had also received some disquieting information from Professor Walter Uphoff, who reported that an article by John Kmetz had appeared in a recent issue of *The Skeptical Inquirer*, which is published by the Committee for the Scientific Investigation into the Claims of the Paranormal. According to Uphoff, this article was 'very one-sided. He takes on the work of Cleve Backster with plants, but is highly selective in the evidence he includes. Kmetz is either ignorant of the work of Marcel Vogel, Paul Savin, Robert Miller and others, or has chosen to ignore their work because it does not fit his conclusions.' Uphoff concluded his letter with: 'I hope that Kmetz will not do a similar job on the experiments in which you participated.'

I wrote to Kmetz and to G.W. Church of the Science Unlimited Research Foundation, which funded the experiments.

I received no reply from either of them and was eventually informed, by Gary Heseltine, a research associate of the Foundation, that Kmetz had left to take up an academic post at Kean College in New Jersey. Then he delivered his bombshell: 'A couple of days after your departure last year,' he wrote, 'it was found that large numbers of cells could be dislodged from the flask by a light finger tap or by properly agitating the flask. Thus the conclusion that a paranormal influence was involved cannot be drawn because of the manner in which the experiments were conducted . . .'

Completely bewildered, I wrote to William Braud, enclosing a copy of Heseltine's letter. Braud's surprise and dismay equalled mine. He replied privately to me and separately sent the following to the *Journal for Psychical Research* in London.

A matter has come to my attention which has relevance to certain statements made in my recent paper in this 'Journal' concerning our work with Matthew Manning. Those statements involved Matthew's work with Dr John Kmetz of Science Unlimited Research Foundation in San Antonio. *I remarked upon Matthew's success in influencing cervical cancer cells in vitro. This I did after witnessing some of the experiments first hand and after Dr Kmetz had supplied me with a copy of the data from the tests done with Matthew.*

I have since learned that some of these results have been called into question because of a recently discovered possible artefact in the experimental protocol.

Kmetz had assured me he had tried a number of physical maneuvers in order to determine whether 'conventional' energy could dislodge the cancer cells from the flask walls, this dislodgement being the target for possible paranormal influences.

He indicated that heat changes, removing the medium from the cells, shaking the flasks, and other physical procedures did not result in the kinds of changes in cell count that resulted from attempts by selected subjects to influence the cells via psychic means. He even indicated that placing the flasks on a vigorous vibrator for some period of time did not dislodge the cells. (I seem to recall that this vibrator was a 'paint shaker', but I'm not certain of this.) *Thus an obvious mechanical artefact would seem to have been ruled out.*

However, we now learn that the cancer cells may be dislodged by dropping the flasks onto a hard surface, abruptly striking the flask with the finger in a certain way, or even vigorously snapping the wrist of the hand holding the flasks. It strikes me as odd that these maneuvers can influence cell counts, while vigorous shaking in a vibrator cannot. It has been suggested that it is the rapid acceleration or 'shock wave' produced by striking that is important. I still wonder about the lack of effect of the starting and stopping acceleration and deceleration of the vibrator. *In any case, because of this possible mechanical artefact, the results of all tests in which flasks are hand-held become suspect. Unfortunately, the majority of Matthew's trials were done under hand-held conditions.*

My own belief is that, although mechanical trauma to hand-held flasks could have dislodged cells in Matthew's tests, this factor alone does not account for the results obtained with them. *I base this conclusion upon two major observations. First, impressive results occurred during test trials in which I myself observed Matthew very closely.*

I was looking carefully for any movements that might disrupt the cells, for this was before I had learned of Kmetz's precautions to test for the influence of mechanical artefacts. I observed absolutely no evidence of mechanical influence of the type which could dislodge the cells during these successful test trials. *I understand that some of Matthew's sessions were videotaped. It*

*should be possible to examine these videotaped records
with care to determine whether any flask movements
occurred during successful sessions.*

*Second, impressive effects continued to occur during
'hands-off' trials in which Matthew had no contact
whatsoever with the flasks. Matthew would point from
a distance at a selected flask (the target for that trial).
Kmetz would then be the only person to handle the
flasks throughout that experiment. Unfortunately, there
were only a small number of such 'hands-off' tests, not
nearly enough for proper statistical analysis.*

*I have described [Kmetz's] experiments in some detail
for fear that he may choose not to publish them. This
would be unfortunate since, with the proper modifica-
tions, they could be extremely useful for the laboratory
investigation of 'paranormal healing' or psychokinetic
influences upon living target systems.*

The *Journal* published this document as an addendum to Braud's
report of the experiments we had conducted together. I heard
nothing further from Kmetz, but in January 1980, a year after the
tests, the *National Enquirer*, to my amazement, carried a story
about the tests and included quotes from him. Braud had been
under the impression that Kmetz had become disenchanted with
the entire set of experiments, and had decided, in Braud's words,
to 'throw out the baby with the bath water'. The quotes from
Kmetz in the *Enquirer* are bafflingly enthusiastic:

If psychic healers can somehow affect how these cells are
growing, they should be able to use the same effect on
people directly. . . . During experiments Manning focussed
his powers on the cells in the flask. The cells attach themselves to the side of the plastic flask but, if they are knocked
loose, they die. . . . 'Just nudging them with your finger
doesn't get them to float free,' said Dr Kmetz. 'The cells are
attached by some electrical energy to the side of the flask.

You have to disrupt that attraction to get them to float free.
Matthew would hold the flask for 10 to 20 minutes or he
would put the flask on the table and just hold his hands
over the top of it for 10 to 20 minutes . . . The cancer cells
were actually being killed by Matthew . . . In at least 60 per
cent of cases, the results were quite significant. Matthew
got those cells to float free. When an individual who was not
a psychic healer tried to do the same thing, we didn't get
anything.

However, perhaps Kmetz also had a conscience, and reckoned
on few of his peers being avid readers of the tabloid *Enquirer*.

＊　＊　＊

Science, it seemed, was not prepared to assist my attempts to
get healing accepted as a valuable health-enhancing tool. In the
UK the opportunities for working at a grass-roots level among the
still to be converted were strictly limited. There was no thriving
night-club circuit which would welcome me, and lecture tours
were not a well-established part of cultural life here. It was not
feasible to import the kind of work I was doing in the States and
earn a living from it.

I received many invitations to address groups in Britain, but
in most cases these offered only expenses and, occasionally, a
tiny fee. More importantly, the people they attracted were not
the ones I was trying to reach, being in the main Spiritualists
who used healing more as proof of the power of spirit guides
from the 'other side' than as a practical aid to well-being.
However, I was reluctant to pass up any opportunity that would
add to my experience and might help to establish me as a healer.
I did not hesitate when I was invited by the 'Institute of Psychic
and Spiritual Technology' to be a presenter in a four-day
symposium.

This organization had been set up and was run by a delightfully eccentric pair of entrepreneurs. Charles Bullen was ex-RAF

with a theatrical flair that had been put to use during wartime, when he had been involved in mounting shows for the Forces. Win Wood was diminutive with a terrier streak of frightening proportions, which had probably served her well during the years she worked for the Gas Board. The Institute had been specializing in organizing resident weekend Spiritualist conferences at Swanwick in Derbyshire, but these were losing them money and they had decided to get a 'name' that could attract an audience.

I was happy to take part in their symposia and in the process put over what the new me consisted of. Charles and Win were sympathetic to my aim of moving more in the direction of healing, having themselves had some experience of it through their involvement with the Spiritualist movement. It was largely due to their efforts that I began to give healing on a one-to-one basis in Britain. The extensive travelling I was doing made it unfeasible for me to establish a healing practice of my own. Win and Charles had large premises in Leicestershire, which they were prepared to let me use two or three days a month, to fit around my tours and other commitments. They offered to set up all the appointments and take care of the administration.

One of my first patients in Leicestershire was Marguerite Otton from Margate in Kent. She had had breast cancer some years previously. She came for healing after a very aggressive secondary bone cancer was diagnosed which was so far advanced as to be thought virtually untreatable. Her surgeon gave her six months to live. The shock of receiving this devastating piece of news sent her into a decline and brought on stomach pains and weight loss. The hormone tablets prescribed by her doctor had such terrible side-effects that she had to stop taking them.

At this point she came to hear about me and began to receive healing regularly: 'He knew exactly where the pain was without being told. I could feel the burning of his hands and I had marks like sunburn on my back afterwards. I was always sick after treatment – it was as if my body was physically ridding itself of the disease.'

Other reactions have been reported by patients, such as severe diarrhoea or profuse sweating. Doctors who are sympathetic to healing have told me that whatever I am doing may be breaking up malignancy so fast that the only way the body has of throwing it out of the system is through these mechanisms.

Marguerite made a steady recovery from day one of receiving healing. The stomach pains disappeared and she put on weight. She has received no orthodox treatment since starting the healing sessions with me. There is no sign of the cancer, a fact that her surgeon, whom she still sees occasionally, cannot explain. He is amazed by her recovery. At the time of writing she is still alive and well.

In addition to enabling me to work on a one-to-one basis, Win and Charles also organized a series of lectures and healing demonstrations around Britain. For the first half of the evening I would talk about what I called oneness and its relevance to our lives. The second half of the evening would be taken up with me giving direct healing to people in the audience.

This idea of connectedness, and our responsibilities to each other and the planet as a whole, remains a central theme of my work. I want people to make the link between how they are, in terms of attitudes and outlook, and the state of their health and that of the people around them.

Lyall Watson expressed this idea rather well in his phrase, 'Every time you mow the grass you shake the cosmos.' I was very impressed with his books – especially *Supernature* and *The Romeo Error* – which provide an intellectual framework for experiences and happenings that mainstream science ignores. On the few occasions I met Watson I felt we were kindred spirits. He was disarmingly unassuming, despite his amazing capacity for retaining information from the most obscure sources. He was like a data base with a soul and profound human intelligence.

My work with Charles and Win was flexible enough to allow me to continue my frequent touring of the US and to build bridges into other countries. In June 1979 I was invited to visit New Zealand by the Spiritualist Church there. This trip was co-sponsored by

Radio Pacific, a fledgling radio station in which the Church had a shareholding. The schedule for my month-long stay included lectures, healing demonstrations, and TV and radio interviews.

One of my first appearances was at the 2,000-seater Auckland Town Hall. Despite heavy plugging by Radio Pacific, several hundred seats were still unsold on the day of my lecture. I went along to the hall early to get the feel of it and found a noisy crowd at the main entrance, waving banners and handing out leaflets. In the US I was getting used to facing protests by Pentecostalists and similar fundamentalist Christian groups, so the presence of these zealots did not worry me unduly. Their banners and placards warned of the perils that would face all those who entered the hall. Their leaflets contained biblical passages which they believed supported their assertion that I was the work of the Devil and that healing was harmful.

All in all these people did a wonderful job of drumming up customers for those few hundred empty seats. Their demonstration brought the traffic in the vicinity of the hall to a halt. In common with most cities in New Zealand, Auckland was not used to major jams. The bewildered motorists wound down their windows and asked the protesters what was going on. Their curiosity must have been piqued when they were told of the imminent appearance in the town hall of the next best thing to Satan. Many of them parked their cars, bought tickets and came in. By the time I began my presentation, every seat in the hall was occupied. Throughout the evening I was aware of distant waves of sound as the protesters outside sang hymns, chanted and apparently tried to exorcize the building of my influence.

The following morning I gave a live radio interview to Gordon Dryden on Radio Pacific. He asked me what I thought of the people who were protesting against me. My response then accords with my view now. I do not care what people think nor do I care whether they believe in what I do. However, merely to condemn me without paying me the courtesy of listening to my ideas and experiencing one of my demonstrations is neither intelligent nor sensible. I would have more respect for the objectors if they would first listen to what I have to say. I concluded with the provocative observation that their attitude smacked of medieval superstition. At this the phone lines to the studio lit up with calls from offended fundamentalists. One youthful-sounding defender of the faith said: 'I was at your meeting last night. I sat with two friends at the back of the hall as far away from you as we could. We spent the evening praying that your miracles wouldn't work, and were left in no doubt that you are the work of the Devil.'

I had a mental picture of this young man, sitting with the Bible on his knees, thumbing through to find appropriate passages to quote at me chapter and verse.

'Why do you call my healings "miracles" if I'm the work of the Devil?' I asked.

After a few moments of silence, he replied: 'We saw that you were dressed completely in black last night. That is the colour of the Devil.'

If my wits had been sharper that morning, I would have asked him how often he had seen a priest wearing any colour other than black!

I have faced similar opposition from religious groups all over the world. In my experience not even the sub-zero temperatures of a Swedish winter will deter them from their mission, although it struck me on that occasion as unfair and unnecessary to involve small babies and bring them along to demonstrate in such conditions. One sentiment that pervades the literature of such groups is an intolerance of non-believers. I am not a Spiritualist, nor do I subscribe to any formal system of religious belief. In the eyes of fundamentalists this lack of Christian credentials seems in itself to be tantamount to aligning oneself with the Devil. If one is not with Christ one is automatically assumed to be against him, or an unwitting vehicle for carrying the innocent away from God and into the clutches of Satan.

The group that had done its best to disrupt my first meeting in Auckland tried even harder the second time round by attempting to break into the meeting. The ushers prevented this, but as a gesture of goodwill three of their number were offered free tickets. These were declined, prompting the manager of the hall to remark that, 'that young man inside is doing more good than that lot out there'. The ordinary people who came to me in New Zealand seemed to benefit from the healing I gave. I received countless reports of people who had attended the public healing demonstrations recording improvements to conditions affecting mobility, such as frozen shoulder, and back and spinal problems. I managed to fit in about 100 people with more serious problems for one-to-one healing. Two letters I found particularly pleasing. This was the text of the first letter.

> On Tuesday, 5th June 1979, I had an appointment with you for healing.
>
> My main problem has been cancer and also a very severe attack of shingles right around my waist on the left side. This was giving me constant pain. I was also very listless and tired, unable to do much work without extreme effort.
>
> After the healing I felt very relaxed, almost as if I was tranquilized. I went home and slept for about two hours and when I awoke, found that the pain from the shingles was completely gone. This has never reoccurred.
>
> After a couple of days I found that I had regained my energy and am now living a normal life without this terrible tiredness. This normal life includes working a forty-hour week with a demanding job.

The second letter read as follows:

> I received healing from you during the morning of June 11th 1979. Prior to healing I had a headache, stiff neck, pains in my hip joints, knees and left leg, proper grouch.
>
> I felt no sensation during healing until you placed your hands around my left knee, which has been rheumatic

ever since I can remember. My knee felt as though a
needle had been pushed thro' it; with difficulty I
restrained myself from booting you! Afterwards my
headaches became more severe, but then during the day
all my aches and pains gradually subsided.

I received an invitation from an unexpected quarter while I was
in New Zealand. One night I got back to where I was staying to
be told that someone from Buckingham Palace had rung wanting
to speak to me. I laughed, thinking my hosts were trying to wind
me up, and went to bed. I got up the following morning and
went out as usual. When I returned to base later that day, I was
given the same message. This time the person from the Palace
had said he would ring back at a designated time and requested
that I make myself available to take his call. I did, and was told
I had been invited to attend a private dinner party to be hosted
by Prince Philip on 10 July at Buckingham Palace.

This dinner was in a sense themed, and given the title
'Supernature'. All of the people present were interested in the
paranormal. Among the guests were Brian Inglis (journalist and
author of, among other titles, *Natural and Supernatural* and
Fringe Medicine), Sir Angus Ogilvy, Dr Lyall Watson (author of
Supernature and one of the gurus of the ecology movement),
Professor John Hasted (a professor of physics and researcher into
the paranormal), Dr Kit Pedlar (former neurosurgeon, author of
the TV series *Doomwatch* and researcher into the paranormal),
Lord Buxton (head of Anglia Television), Professor Lord
Zuckerman (zoologist and educationalist), Rev. Martin Israel (an
authority on exorcism) and Sir John Whitmore (philanthropist
and patron of psychic research).

On my right sat Earl Mountbatten, and on my left Sebastian
de Ferranti, Chairman of Ferranti Limited. I wondered if I might
be in for a repeat of the experience with Lord Rothschild, but
Mr Ferranti seemed genuinely interested in my abilitites. Earl
Mountbatten talked a great deal about reincarnation, in which
he believed unhesitatingly, and was convinced that his late

wife, Edwina, had communicated with him since her death. Five weeks later he would be murdered by the IRA.

One of the topics of conversation around the table was whether psychokinetic energy could be put to positive use. I told them about my experience of healing. Sir Angus Ogilvy was particularly well informed and had heard about my experiments in Texas with both cancer and blood cells. He was enthusiastic about the possibilities and was confident that his contacts with BUPA and the Imperial Cancer Research Fund, of which he was Chairman, could be put to good use. The strength of his enthusiasm worried Brian Inglis, who was afraid that too close an association with an endeavour to get healing off the ground might damage his reputation. What Ogilvy envisaged was, in fact, very sensible: a pilot study into the efficacy of healing, involving people rather than test tubes. As I had been successful in treating both cancer and blood cells, I proposed that I give direct healing to leukaemia patients.

With the disappointment of the Kmetz affair still in my mind, I must confess to being dubious as to whether Ogilvy would be as good as his word and carry the proposal forward. He was, and a group of doctors, led by Professor Hobbs at the Royal Free Hospital in London, set about trying to establish a protocol for the study. Unfortunately, that was as far as we got. In its capacity as the medical profession's insurance company the Medical Defence Union (MDU) raised objections on the grounds that the subject was 'too emotive' and that the tabloid press would have a field day at the doctors' expense if they got hold of the story.

How the MDU came to hear of the experiment is anyone's guess. Mine is that a none too sympathetic doctor tipped them off. In those days the medical profession could be relied upon to be unsympathetic to the point of hostility against this sort of work. With their insurers warning them off, the doctors withdrew their support and the project died a death. Something was salvaged from the wreckage, in the form of an experiment involving intractable pain. The MDU had no problems with this.

The subject of intractable pain may have been close to

Ogilvy's heart because of a persistent back problem of his own. I treated him for this on a number of occasions while the pilot study was in progress, sometimes at the offices of auctioneers Sotheby's, of which he was a director. I did not succeed in curing him, although he expressed his gratitude for being in 'much less pain'. Prince Philip expressed interest in receiving healing for his wrist, which he swore was giving him trouble because of the number of hands he had shaken. His passion for playing polo was a more likely culprit. Later, I believe electro-acupuncture brought him some relief.

Ogilvy's second proposal was called Project Aesculapius – after Aesculapius, or Asclepius, the son of Apollo and Coronis and the god of healing in classical mythology – and was, I believe, the first experiment of its kind in Britain. Professor Hobbs was, again, designated as the project leader. He was open-minded about healing, simply because a patient of his with liver disease had got better as a result of receiving it from the renowned Harry Edwards. He told me: 'As a doctor I simply can't explain what happened, but I've never forgotten it.'

The project was funded by the Koestler Foundation. (The Foundation was unique in its remit: to support and finance research into phenomena which do not fit a regular scientific structure and cannot be explained in materialist terms.) Eight patients from the Royal Free's Pain Clinic took part in the experiment, which ran from April to September 1980. They were told that they had a 50:50 chance of receiving healing from me. I was the only person who knew to which patients treatment was being given.

The preliminary results showed that the patients who wanted the treatment and with whom I felt I had established a good rapport experienced less pain and/or were able to reduce their intake of drugs. This was the case whether or not I treated them. The doctors explained the results in terms of cognitive dissonance theory, which broadly means that because the patients felt involved in their treatment, they were more inclined to believe it was working, and therefore it was more likely to work. This has become one the medical profession's favourite ways of dismissing healing. Whenever I hear it, I think of a small wire-haired Dachshund called Barney, who surely goes some way towards disproving this theory!

Barney belonged to Marguerite Otton, one of my patients. He, like other standard Dachshunds, had a weak back because of the practice of interbreeding to produce longer 'sausage dogs'. In March 1985 the seven-year-old Barney had jumped off a wall, injuring his back so badly that he was left incontinent and with both back legs paralysed. He was game enough to insist on getting around by using his front legs to drag himself along.

An X-ray of Barney's back showed, according to the vet's report, 'a Class 4 disc protrusion at the thoraco-lumbar junction'. The pressure on the spinal cord from this protrusion was causing the paralysis and the incontinence. The extent of the damage to Barney's spine was such that the vet considered him 'not a suitable candidate for de-compression surgery'. Regretfully, he advised Marguerite to have Barney put down. She was torn, loving the dog and yet not wanting to see him in pain. I remember her calling and asking if she could bring Barney with her to our next healing session which, as luck would have it, was scheduled for the following day.

I can still recall that session quite clearly, and see Barney lying on a towel in her lap. Marguerite had cancer in her spine and I spent the whole session directing my energy to that area of her body. I did not think about Barney, nor did I place my hands on him at any time. At the end of the healing she took him home, still paralysed.

When she came downstairs the following morning and went into the kitchen, she was astonished to be greeted by Barney running round and round the kitchen in circles wagging his tail. She made another appointment with the vet to have Barney X-rayed again. Sure enough the dog's back showed no injury. The vet was completely baffled and had no explanation for what had happened. Barney suffered no further problems with his back, as the vet, G.J.G. Shawcross, would confirm in a letter to me later:

I had the opportunity to see Barney at intervals until 25 April 1988 when he was euthanazed for an unrelated problem.

During the three years following my initial assessment, his hind legs and bladder function made an almost perfect recovery.

Barney cannot be said to have had faith in healing; nor can what happened be explained in terms of placebo effect or psychological factors.

What occurred in the case of Simon Acherman, a six-year-old autistic child who was brought to me when I visited Switzerland in 1980, is equally difficult to explain in terms of cognitive dissonance. The child's mother reported:

> Before healing, his eyes rolled uncontrollably, he couldn't speak properly and rarely answered questions. After one session there was immediate benefit. His eyes no longer rolled and he could focus. He followed conversations and answered questions intelligently. It is a remarkable healing that has even surprised the child's therapists.

Is a child with such problems really going to derive benefit solely as a result of psychological factors?

Project Aesculapius was not a satisfactory endeavour from my perspective, because the measure of success was so imprecise. The first proposal would at least have allowed blood cells to be counted. Pain is a subjective phenomenon. It cannot be measured, and the results of the trial were dependent too much on the patients themselves. For example, occasionally a patient would report feeling better but would fail to register this in the so-called 'pain scale' which he or she was asked to complete at the end of each week.

There were other problems associated with the experiment. In some patients it was thought that addiction meant their intake of drugs was not necessarily related to their level of pain. In other patients closed-mindedness was observed which, it was felt, made them unable to provide feedback on their levels of pain after receiving treatment from me.

I have not been invited back to the Palace since that dinner. This cannot be because my table manners were not good enough. At the end of the meal, one of the liveried waiters brought out a huge gold bowl piled high with fruit. Because I was rather nervous I did not take time to choose, but stuck my hand into the pile and pulled out what was there.

When I looked at my catch, I discovered with horror that I had landed a handful of cherries. What, I wondered, is the correct way of eating them in these august surroundings? I was sure that some protocol concerning the pips must have been devised. Then I noticed that Prince Philip, who was sitting across the table from me, also had cherries on his plate. I decided to watch what he did. To my amusement, he spat the cherry stones straight out of his mouth onto the plate in front of him. My usual method is preferable to that, I thought, and got on with eating.

Professor John Hasted was one of the few dinner guests at Buckingham Palace that evening whom I had met before. He had conducted a test with me earlier in the year at Birkbeck College in which I had tried to influence the growth rate of moulds; this was the final test in the series done under the auspices of the London Society for Psychical Research. In 1980 we came across each other again, when he assisted American neurochemist Professor Glen Rein in a series of experiments designed to gauge whether psychokinetic energy could affect the metabolism of neurotransmitters, and specifically the enzyme monoamine oxydase (MAO). This enzyme was still a relatively unknown entity, having only recently (the early 1970s) been discovered in the blood in the brain by US neurochemists.

Glen Rein was doing research at Queen Charlotte's Hospital in London to find out why women who suffer from migraines tend not to get them when they are pregnant. He was following up an observation made by the researchers who had originally identified monoamine oxydase, that there might be a link between the level of MAO in the brain and migraines. The researchers noted that the level of this enzyme in the brain dropped just before the onset of a migraine. However, they were not sure whether the migraine was causing the drop in the enzyme level or the decrease in the enzyme was causing the migraine.

Rein had a personal interest in healing and he wanted to find out if it could influence MAO. He reasoned that if an influence could be demonstrated with the enzyme in a test tube, healing should be able to bring relief to actual migraine sufferers. I was asked to try to increase the activity of the enzyme. According to Rein this would be harder to achieve than the reverse because 'it is likely to be easier to cause a (negative) change in the direction the system is already going, e.g. to increase degradation.'

The results of this experiment proved difficult to explain. After receiving healing from me, the enzyme increased or decreased its activity by as much as 40 per cent. In nine of the trials the activity of the enzyme increased (in some trials quadrupling), in seven of them activity decreased, and in two of the trials the enzyme level did not change relative to the test tubes of blood cells I did not treat. Rein thought it 'remarkable' that I should be able to reverse the system's natural tendency.

Glen Rein was a most unusual scientist. I came to the conclusion that his primary purpose in doing the experiment with me was so he could learn how to develop as a healer himself. He had some very strong ideas on how the qualities required for healing might be enhanced, and had imposed on himself a very long list of prohibitions.

Anything that might upset his nervous system was forbidden – alcohol, tobacco, illegal substances and the many foods not included in the strict vegan's diet sheet. During the lunch break he would always use two ionizers to clear the air in the laboratory, because he thought the right ions might make the results even better. He also brought in his own packed lunch of macrobiotic goodies. I took myself off to a nearby pub for a pint of beer. One day he forgot his lunch and I suggested, partly in jest, that he come with me. His face dropped when I told him where I went.

I am not sure whether he was disappointed in me or whether I had presented him with an unexpected dilemma, in that although he wanted my company he was concerned that venturing across the threshold of such a place might endanger his dream of becoming a healer. I tried to ease his dilemma, impressing upon him that he could have bottled water or a soft drink and a sandwich. Very reluctantly, he agreed to come with me. At the pub I ordered a pint of Guinness and took it to the table where he was sitting. He looked at it disapprovingly, but said nothing. It was a very hot day and I was soon ready for another pint. When I came back with my second Guinness and put it on the table, he could not contain himself:

'You're not going to drink that one as well, are you?'

I said, 'Well, I'm certainly not going to leave it there. I've just bought it.'

'But you'll wreck the experiments. You won't be able to do anything.'

I did not like to tell him that this lunchtime was no different to any other and that on each of the other experiment days I had returned to the laboratory fortified by a couple of decent pints of Guinness. Later, when he came to analyse the results of the trials, it became very apparent that all the experiments conducted in the afternoons yielded results that were statistically more significant than those done in the mornings. Contrary to what he had supposed, the Guinness had obviously helped my performance, probably because it had relaxed me.

In addition to Project Aesculapius one other experiment came out of that evening at Buckingham Palace. I was invited to appear in a programme presented by Dr Kit Pedlar to see if I could replicate the cancer-cell experiment I had done with Kmetz. Pedlar was a sort of gamekeeper turned poacher, in that he had once been part of the medical establishment and had given up his career as a

neurosurgeon to pursue a greater interest in alternative medicine
and in the role of mind over matter in questions of health.

I was unsure what difference the presence of television
cameras might make to the dynamics of what I was attempting.
I did not fully understand how my healing abilities worked, or
why they could not be relied upon to be successful 100 per cent
of the time. Here I was agreeing to put myself on the line in the
most public way imaginable. I felt I had no option. I wanted to
show that the Kmetz experiments had not been flawed, and that
healing was valid in terms that ordinary people, as well as scientists, would be able to understand. Kit Pedlar's attitude helped to
create a positive atmosphere in that most unnatural of environ-
ments, and for the duration of the experiment I managed to
forget where I was.

Hela cervical cancer cells were again used, and put into three
plastic flasks. I tried to influence one flask, Dr Pedlar (who
claimed to have no healing powers) tried to do the same with
another and the third received no treatment from either of us.
Under the glare of the TV lights, I tried to heal the cells. After the
experiment the contents of the three flasks were inspected with
an electrospectrograph, then Dr Pedlar gave the result. The
readings in the flask exposed to Dr Pedlar and in the control
flask were identical within experimental error. The number of
dead cells in the flask exposed to me was 20 per cent higher
than in either of the other flasks, a fact which, as Dr Pedlar said
at the time, 'tends to confirm what [was] achieved in 27 out of 30
trials in America'.

This experiment drew a line under my relationship with test
tubes. They no longer seemed important. I had proved all I was
capable of proving with them. One certainty I took away from
the intractable pain experiment at the Royal Free is that healing
is a two-way activity in which the patient participates. This participation may be on a level he or she does not fully understand
or is not even aware of.

It may be that those patients to whom I was not ostensibly
giving treatment but who wanted healing to help them were, in

fact, healing themselves. If, as I believe, each of us possesses innate healing abilities, it follows that these can be used to keep us well and help us to overcome specific health problems. You do not have to believe in healing for it to work. Essential, though, is a strong desire to get better.

A positive state of mind is a potent tool for healing, and one I use all the time. When I give healing, I expect to achieve a good result. I expect the people I treat to be active partners. When I first began to give healing, this was a novel idea that took some grasping. Many people who came to me were used to being the passive recipients of 'health care'. One of my earliest 'messages' was, 'You are your own best healer,' and this was the theme of many of my talks and demonstrations. I would teach simple meditation and visualization techniques to get people used to this way of working. Soon people were telling me how helpful they were, and it seemed a good idea to record them on to tape so that people could create a healing ambience in their own homes. A cassette tape, called *Healing and Self-healing*, was the first of many. Producing it forced me to confront a problem I had been trying to ignore for several years.

Cassette tapes were the only form of media not covered by the contract I had signed with Peter Bander's company, Van Duren Publications, shortly before publication of *The Link*. As far as the rest went, I seemed to be tied up for life, with Van Duren legally entitled to half the proceeds from any future television work, film rights, book or article. I had signed that contract blind, without receiving the benefit of independent legal advice. My father had looked at the original contract with Colin Smythe Limited, and I think we both assumed the terms of the second contract would be identical, except for the change in company names.

Brian Inglis urged me to do something about the contract. Earlier he had encouraged me to get away from Peter Bander and make my own career. He had been right in that regard and I knew he was right now. His argument was irrefutable: I could find myself in a situation where I was forced to part with money that I had earned by my own efforts without any help from Bander.

In addition to Brian's invaluable support, I was fortunate in having the friendship of Instone Bloomfield. As a high-powered financier, dealing with money and what makes it work was his business. On a personal level he had a deep interest in psychical research and spirituality. I have never had a head for business, and it was not a topic of the many conversations we had. Like Brian, who was a close friend, he took a benevolent interest in me and what I was up to. This extended from giving friendly advice to funding the experiments with the SPR. He knew those experiments were important to me and with a few strokes of a pen he had made them possible.

After studying my contract with Bander, Bloomfield told me that I would have to go to court if I wanted to extricate myself. My heart sank. I had put off doing anything about the contract precisely because I did not want to get involved in some legal wrangle. Then he said: 'If you want to sue Bander, I'll back you. If you win, great. If you don't, it doesn't matter. I don't want the money back.'

Disquieting information emerged during the months it took to put together the case against Bander. A director who had signed the contract for *In the Minds of Millions* on behalf of W.H. Allen told me that his company had bought world rights from Van Duren, based on the success of *The Link*, and had lost heavily on the deal when the sales failed to live up to their much-hyped expectations. The story I had got from Peter Bander at the time was that he had sold only UK rights on the book. Shortly after signing this contract, Bander had bought another house in Gerrards Cross.

I have never seen the difference between the monies received by Van Duren for UK and world rights. I am sure they would have amounted to more than the £1,500 passed on to me. I discovered, too, that Van Duren were unusual among publishers in deducting all their running costs and expenses from my share of monies received. These deductions were hefty, and pruned substantial amounts from my originally healthy looking 60 per cent share. The biggest cheek had been Bander making me a 'director' of Van Duren Publications and giving me one share in the company. At the time my 'elevation' was cited as proof of Bander's fair dealing. I did not need that director, who had by this time left W.H. Allen and fallen out with Bander, to tell me that I had been taken for a ride, but he did anyway.

In the end, Bander settled out of court, and I was released from all contractual ties. I had regained my freedom.

*　　*　　*

The United States was the one place I repeatedly escaped to while this legal drama played itself out. There were always towns I had not visited. My opportunities in the States widened still further when I was taken up by Silva Mind Control. This opening had come through Gerry Seavey, who organized many of my first US tours and was an instructor in the Silva Method, which shows people how to achieve dynamic mental skills through stress management and deep-relaxation techniques.

This course had been devised by José Silva, an electronics engineer from Laredo, Texas, in 1966 after twenty years of research. His method teaches people to create a balance between the right and left sides of the brain and through this balance to become more successful in all areas of their lives. The Silva Method has often been called a course in positive thinking, but Silva himself described his techniques as holistic and his aim is for people to become positive beings, not merely positive thinkers. Essentially, his message is one that most people would subscribe to: that we function better at all levels when we are fully relaxed mentally and physically.

By the time I became aware of the Silva Method it was established as the Western pioneer of mind-development programmes, with several million graduates. Representatives of Silva Mind Control asked me to do workshops on psychic development, a facility which they considered to be essential for better awareness and decision making. Although I had not done their course, the organization accepted me as one of its own, because there was so much overlap between our material.

What I was doing was complementary to the Silva Method in that I seemed to be confirming José Silva's teachings and taking people one stage on from what was termed their Graduate's Course. The organization's large mailing list guaranteed me an audience of hundreds wherever I visited under the Silva banner. Even some night-clubs in the States were running Silva courses to increase their takings. One club owner in Denver had managed to treble his turnover, and he planned to do the same in a club he owned in the Rockies. He asked me to give a healing demonstration there, which I did. The mountain men who had made that area their own as the United States carved out its identity could not have been a harder audience to crack.

The Silva organization enabled me to reach a wider audience than ever before, and because of its backing my name and face became increasingly well known in the States. I was pleased when José Silva himself asked me if I would like to lecture and give healing demonstrations in Rio de Janeiro in August 1980. I looked on this trip as an education. I loved the idea of going to South America, and especially to Brazil, which has a long tradition of healing.

The Brazilian spiritual psyche could be said to be split between Roman Catholicism, the predominant religion, and the animist beliefs of its native Indian population. The attitude towards healing is one of acceptance. In Brazil there exists a kind of coalition between the Church and the native medicine men, with each side of the spiritual divide appreciating the contribution of the other. I felt a little bit presumptuous, bringing my meagre experience to this Mecca of healing and psychic surgery.

I was overwhelmed by the generosity of the Brazilian people and their willingness to accept me. Some 2,000 people turned up to see me, one of the largest audiences I had ever had. The demonstration went very well – people who had not been able to bend for years were touching their toes and saying they were free of pain. When the effect of the healing became clear to the audience, there was uproar.

I had never been the recipient of such enthusiasm. There was so much, it was frightening. People were storming the stage, trying to get hold of me. I managed to get off before my clothes were ripped from my back, and eventually escaped to my hotel. I then became a virtual prisoner for three days, as a succession of people wanting to see me crowded into the hotel foyer. Some of them even tried to get up to my room. Eventually they drifted away and I was left in peace, but it was one of the few times I felt endangered.

After Brazil I revisited New Zealand to give workshops on how to heal. As on my previous visit, I put time aside to see people on a one-to-one basis. Leo Ross Forbes was among the many people who made appointments with me. He was only forty-five, and suffering from both arthritis and a condition called Huntington's Chorea, a hereditary disease characterized by chronic, progressive and involuntary twitching of the muscles and dementia. The cause of the disease is unknown and, according to textbooks in orthodox medicine, there is no effective treatment.

Leo's balance was affected by the disease, which meant he had great difficulty walking straight. After receiving healing, he wrote to me:

I was never very sure of my footsteps. In the last three years I had lost all sense of taste and smell. After the first treatment with you my whole body flowed day and night with a wonderful warmth, and even though it was mid-winter I found that I didn't need my electric blanket, despite the fact that I had been using it every night for the previous two months.

Immediately 70 per cent of my arthritic pains left me. The Huntington's Chorea improved straight away. I could walk much more steadily and 80 per cent of my ability to smell returned with a bang. For the first time in three years I could actually taste my food. After the third treatment I improved even more. The Huntington's Chorea, which caused me so much trouble, has practically gone. I can speak more easily and my arthritis is 90 per cent improved. I am not dragging myself about any more. I am full of beans. You have changed my life completely. I feel wonderful all over. Life is beautiful again.

The Swiss received me with rather more restraint when I toured their country for a month in the summer of 1980, giving public demonstrations in Zürich, Lugano, Berne, Lucerne and Stans. Among the several children brought to me by desperate parents was eight-year-old Claude Fontana, who had no bladder control day or night. After one treatment this problem was resolved.

Heinz Suter, a busy executive in his late forties, from Oberentfelden, Aarau, wrote to me in April 1981 about his experience of the demonstration he had attended. In October 1979 he had visited his family doctor complaining of continuous pain and bowel cramps. The doctor discovered a fissure caused by a growth and referred him to a specialist. Heinz was informed that the growth was malignant and that major surgery was the only advisable course of action. He did not relish this prospect and, in spite of pain and an almost constant high temperature, attempted to continue living as normally as possible. Then he heard that I was to give a workshop in Zürich and made an appointment to receive treatment.

'The healing was given to me at midday, and eighteen hours later I had no more pain,' he wrote. In April the following year Heinz plucked up courage to go back to the specialist for a re-examination. No trace could be found of the fissure or of the growth in Heinz's bowel. 'After that sudden, unexpected healing I was given a new perspective to life. What I received was something very precious.'

Six months after the Swiss tour, I was invited by the German magazine *Esotera* to give lectures and demonstrations in Munich,

Freiburg, Karlsruhe, Stuttgart, Düsseldorf and Bremen. Doctors and journalists were among the 450 people drawn to the first meeting, at the Penta Hotel in Munich. I had learned from my experiences in the 1970s that the German media are just about the most cynical in Europe, so I was expecting negative coverage.

Among the volunteers I treated from the audience were a young woman who had been deaf in her left ear for three months, and sixty-two-year-old Lisa who was unable to raise her arms because of arthritis. After healing, the young woman could again hear the jangling of coins and clicking of fingernails some distance from the ear. Her hearing was still not 100 per cent, but it was much improved. One of the doctors present called this spontaneous result 'amazing'. At the end of her session with me, Lisa said that she felt as though her whole body had been harmonized. She then lifted both arms high above her head and shouted, 'They work again!'

The following morning the German daily *Bild-Zeitung* described the healings as miracles and quoted one of the doctors who had witnessed the results. He was referred to only as Dr Hans Christian Sch, to protect his reputation. 'Orthodox doctors and scientists are not yet sufficiently open to the possibilities of such healing,' he declared. He was so impressed by what he saw that later he came to watch me treat twenty-six people privately.

Other eminent doctors who made themselves known to me during this trip echoed this concern about the attitude of many of their fellows. In Stuttgart a cancer specialist, Professor Heinkel, invited me to visit his research laboratory, where we discussed healing. He believed that many doctors needed to learn to relate to their patients as human beings. The tendency, he thought, was to regard sick people as one might a broken-down car.

After the report in *Bild-Zeitung* I was virtually besieged in my hotel. I treated as many people as I could in the short time available to me. Shortly before I left Bavaria I received a warning that I was in danger of being arrested. I did not take this too seriously. I was leaving for Freiburg, in the neighbouring *Land* of Baden-Württemberg, and was intent on encouraging the doctors who were now coming to watch me work to check people before and after I gave healing.

Two of the doctors present at my first demonstration in Freiburg verified that the arms of Friedrich Landenberger were locked and that the osteoarthritis from which he had suffered for years prevented him from raising them above shoulder height. After treatment his pain vanished, and he could lift his arms above his head. There to witness and record the scene was an array of reporters and photographers. 'Before' and 'after' photographs of Herr Landenberger subsequently appeared in magazines across Europe.

The most dramatic healing effected on that occasion involved Frau Ripprich, the wife of one of the doctors present. Dr Ripprich explained to the audience that his wife had injured her right elbow over a year ago and was unable to straighten her arm; any attempt to do so caused her considerable pain. Another doctor was asked to examine Frau Ripprich before I gave healing. After five minutes of treatment, Frau Ripprich could straighten her arm without pain.

Manfred Seng of Fulda was one of the people I treated privately during my stay in Freiburg. In the latter half of 1980 he had developed a persistent cough that did not respond to any of the medications prescribed by his doctor. After three months his symptoms also included severe weight loss and night sweats.

In April 1981 Manfred was sent to his local hospital for tests. These revealed a tumour between the heart and lung which, according to Manfred, was 'the size of a child's head'. In addition to this fast-growing Morbus Hodgkin, another tumour was found in his liver. He had also developed jaundice. His consultant held out little hope: 'He came to me and told me, in the presence of other patients, that I could consult ten other professors but they would all tell me the same: I would not see the end of the year. Now I was totally dispirited.' Manfred was referred to Professor Mussow in Baden-Baden, a leading cancer specialist, who immediately booked a bed for him in the University Clinic in Freiburg.

When I first treated Manfred, he had no appetite, his cough

was continuous and the night sweats were so heavy that his mattress had to be changed regularly. The cancer, he had been told, was now in secondary stages.

'After the first sessions with you, things began to improve,' he wrote to me later. 'My appetite came back and I was even able to eat breakfast with other patients on the ward. The doctors were very surprised.'

A year later Manfred was still alive and 'all the doctors can do is wonder about my great improvement'. I treated him on two or three further occasions, in 1982, until I felt he did not need my help any more. In 1984 he sent his mother, Regina, to me after she was diagnosed with malignant polyps in her colon. She had several healing sessions with me in England before undergoing surgery in Cologne. The surgeon who operated on her was surprised when no traces of malignancy could be found.

Manfred made a full recovery and over ten years later he assured me he was still fit and healthy. At the time of writing, he is still referring cases to me.

The last stop on my tour was the northern German city-state of Bremen. Representatives of one of the largest German press agencies came to my demonstration there, accompanied by five doctors who had been invited to attend as witnesses. One of these doctors, leading orthopaedic surgeon Dr Thomas Hansen, was particularly impressed by the effect of healing on a patient with an arthritic shoulder. The following day Dr Hansen reported that the amazement of watching her move her arm, without pain, in all directions, had prevented him from sleeping a wink. He said that the orthodox method of treatment would have involved giving an anaesthetic to enable him to move the arm – which he said would be like 'breaking concrete' – followed by several weeks of physiotherapy to restore full movement. 'Yet Matthew Manning can do this in ten minutes,' he exclaimed. Several people I treated privately while in Bremen were sent to me by their doctors.

I flew home, pleased that the trip had gone so well and that I had been invited to return. I did not realize that I was a marked man in the eyes of the German authorities. In those days I took healing to every country where an opening presented itself. I did not concern myself with finding out about the laws. If people were prepared to invite me, I would go. In Britain we have laws that tell us what we cannot do. In Germany, it seems, laws tell them what they can do. There is no law legalizing healing, therefore it is illegal. There are healers in Germany, but they work very unobtrusively, so as not to attract the attention of the authorities.

When I touched down in Munich again a few months later, the organizer of the lecture I was to give informed me that a sympathetic doctor had warned him that I should not attempt to give any public healing during the lecture because the authorities were watching me.

During the course of the lecture it became apparent who their agents were. While I was talking about self-healing, relaxation and meditation, my attention was repeatedly drawn to three men in the audience. They were clearly not riveted by my presentation, exuding scepticism, whispering together and taking notes. At the end of the lecture they rifled through the literature and tapes on display, before coming over to where I was standing with the organizer and introducing themselves.

One was a doctor, one a police officer and another a government official. What these three had witnessed had not contravened German law. However, it was made absolutely clear that if I had so much as placed my hands on somebody, the papers carried by the government official would have been served immediately and I would have been arrested for practising medicine without a licence. If I had done a basic one year's training in Germany and received a certificate which said I was a Heilpraktiker, or health practitioner, I would have been safe from prosecution.

Practising openly in Germany was very difficult for me after this experience. Wherever I went in the country I felt under constant threat, looking over my shoulder all the time to check that I was not being watched. Much the same feeling of unease and wariness eventually accompanied me to France, where healing is also illegal.

Encouraged by the success of my first trip there, I risked giving public healing demonstrations until it became obvious that to continue to do so would land me in trouble with the authorities. On my last visit I was forced to leave the country more quickly than I had planned to in order to avoid being arrested by the police. Fortunately, neither the German nor the French authorities could stop their citizens from voting with their feet and receiving healing from me in England.

To add to the uncertainty, I discovered that a distinction had to be made between laws and attitudes to laws. Healing is technically illegal in Switzerland, but I have never experienced a problem with the Swiss authorities. The Swiss are often characterized as being conformist busy-bodies with a law for everything. When it comes to healing, though, even their officials are laid back and accepting.

In Britain healing has been legal for over fifty years and before that it had a long tradition. It was somewhat ironic, therefore, that of all the countries I had visited as a healer, I should be struggling to establish my credentials in Britain. I attributed this situation to the way I was working. Both Charles and Win were what I call music-hall Spiritualists and many of the venues we worked as a team attracted the sort of people who regularly attend Spiritualist Church 'services'.

I would look out from the platform at rows of elderly people, many of whom regarded healing as something being done to them by agents from the 'other side' working through the healer. Their minds were completely fixed about the nature of healing and its processes. I was not sure how it worked, but they were in no doubt. Some of them would become very irritated with me when I tried to put across my ideas about self-healing and the importance of making healing part of our everyday lives. Concern for the environment, developing awareness, and taking time for meditation and creative visualization were irrelevant to them and to their concept of healing. I remember at one of my early workshops an old man struggling to his feet, waving his walking stick at me and shouting: 'Keep to the healing, boy!'

That was the dismaying message I was receiving from all around me. Much of the problem could be put down to the generation gap existing between me and the people attending these public demonstrations. I sensed the atmosphere of a time-warp, of not being able to consider anything different because of an almost umbilical attachment to what is known and understood. It was worlds away from what I was encountering in the States and elsewhere outside Britain, where I was attracting genuine cross-sections of the communities I visited. Although Win and Charles were happy to continue along the lines they had laid for themselves years previously, I was not. My route had to be one that reached the widest audience.

*   *   *

I had met Graham Wilson in 1978 when he had invited me to lecture at his Festival for Mind, Body and Spirit in London. Graham was a pioneer and his aim for the Festival was to bring the alternative lifestyle options exhibited at the Festival into the mainstream, so they were no longer restricted to narrow cliques. We were kindred souls. He had always had an interest in alternative lifestyles and had worked extensively on self-empowerment courses in the States.

When I decided to strike out on my own, without Win and Charles, Graham was the first person with whom I discussed my options. I wanted to repeat in Britain the success of my tours in the United States, New Zealand, Germany and elsewhere. Together Graham and I organized a tour of lectures and demonstrations that would take place in eleven towns and cities across the country in July 1981. We were equal partners in the enterprise, agreeing to share any profits or losses.

As I was aiming to attract a wider, younger audience, I decided to try to 'package' myself and so give my presentation extra 'edge'. I did not want anyone mistaking me for that naive, shy 'Poltergeist

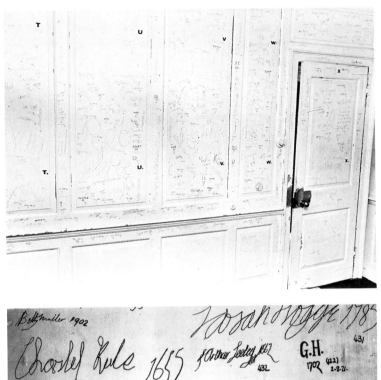

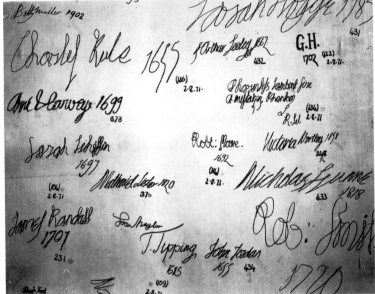

The 'spirit graffiti' of Queen's House: 503 signatures, with dates, appeared on the walls in my bedroom between 31 July and 6 August 1971. Many of the names were those of local families and in some cases the accompanying dates were those on which the named persons died. (Vernon Harrison)

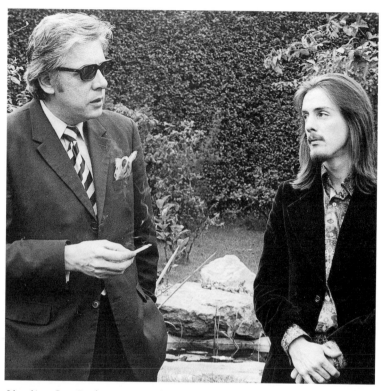

Listening to Peter Bander, my manager from 1973 to 1977.

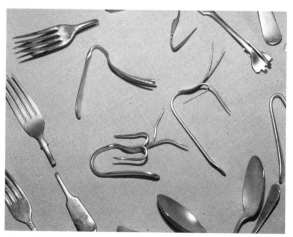

An assortment of
the cutlery which I
broke or bent
during my visit to
Toronto in June
1974. I was there
to participate in a
series of experiments
which were to form
the basis of the first
Canadian conference
on psychokinesis.

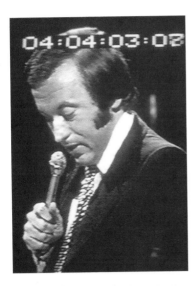

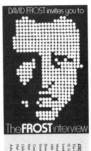

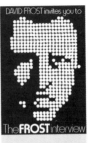

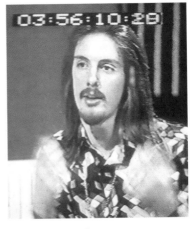

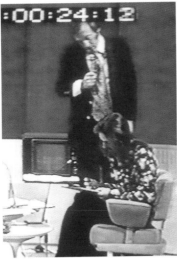

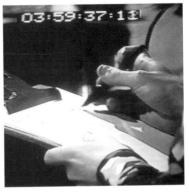

My first exposure to the mainstream media –
appearing on BBC Television's *The Frost
Interview* in October 1974 to talk about my
experiences and demonstrate automatic
writing. David Frost was said to have been
'reduced to a quivering jelly'. That made two
of us.   (BBC Television)

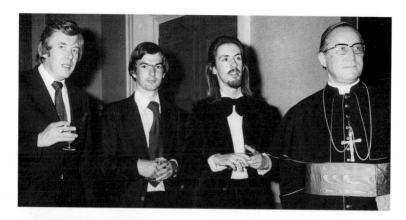

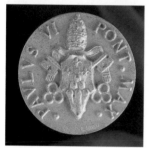

'There was no psychic consultation.' – Archbishop.
Here I am, accompanied by Peter Bander and Leslie
Hayward, at the London home of Archbishop Bruno
Heim, who was then the Vatican's ambassador to
Britain. Left is the Papal medal I was given as thanks
for a diagnosis I provided, through automatic writing,
for Pope Paul VI.

This cartoon sums up the general view of me projected
by the media.   (Colin Smythe Ltd.)

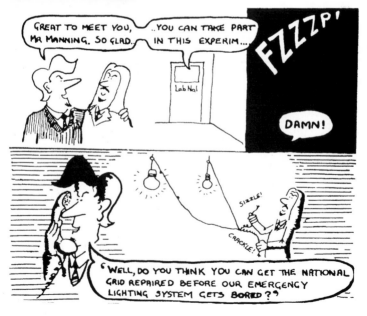

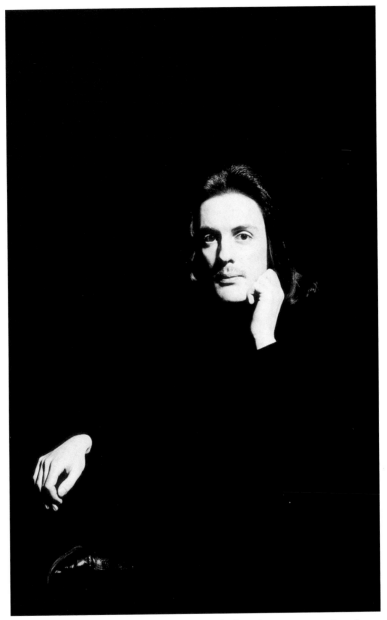

A studio portrait by Snowdon, taken for Vogue magazine in 1978 to accompany an interview. (Condé Nast Publications)

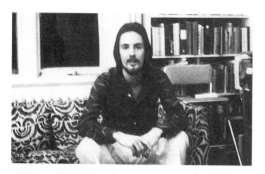
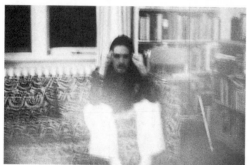
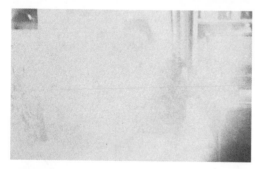
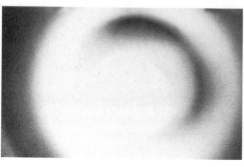

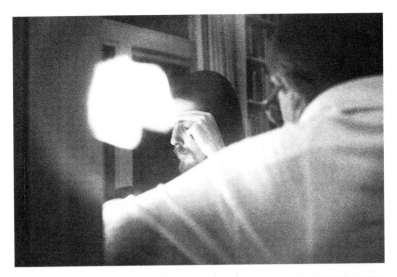

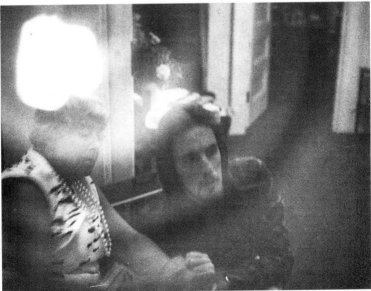

A series of polaroid photographs taken during my stay with Professor George Owen and his wife, Iris, in autumn 1977. The first image, on the left-hand page, is a perfectly normal shot of me looking into the camera lens. In the second shot mistiness is forming around me as I begin to meditate and feel tingling in my hands. By frame four white concentric rings of light have virtually obscured everything in the room, including me. While the polaroids above were being taken, I was trying first to visualize a ball of light coming from my head and then to transfer the energy to Iris.

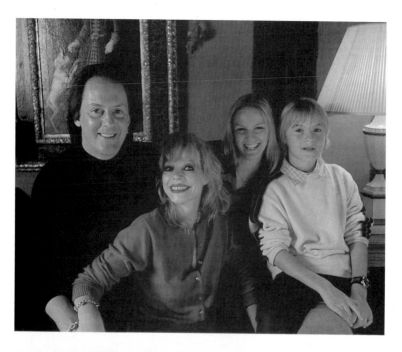

Above: Gig, Henrietta,
Jethro and I: 2003.

Left: Healing.

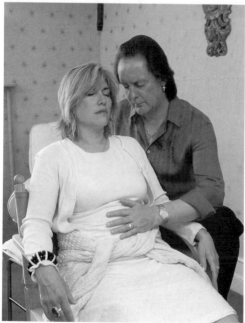

Boy'. This was to be new-style rather than New Age healing, assisted by a large set decorated in shades of blue, a backdrop onto which mood slides could be projected, and Pink Floyd decibelling out of the sound system. It was rather showbiz, rather different, and not calculated to draw Spiritualist Church goers.

The first venue was London's Olympia Exhibition Centre, where I gave a demonstration as part of Graham's Festival of Mind, Body and Spirit. It was a good way of getting publicity for the tour, which was not scheduled to start in earnest until 8 July.

Among the several people I selected for treatment was the BBC Radio London personality Colin Maitland. He had lost his sense of smell sixteen years previously as a result of fracturing his skull in an accident. He had consulted specialists in Harley Street without success. I gave him healing for several minutes and then handed him three small bottles to see if he could tell their contents apart by smell. He did not react at all when he sniffed at the first two bottles, the one containing aftershave and the other diluted smelling salts. When he snorted at the contents of the third bottle, he recoiled sharply and pulled a face. Minutes after leaving the platform he could still smell the methylated spirits in that bottle.

I was sure I could help Colin further and when the *News of the World* newspaper expressed interest in organizing an experiment to test my healing powers, I suggested that he might like to be included among the twelve people they proposed should be selected. Each of the twelve would have two private healing sessions with me. The paper arranged for two doctors to be on hand to witness the healing and to comment on the results. At the end of our session, Colin was able to smell vinegar and smelling salts.

Len Shorter of the north London suburb of Palmers Green arrived for his session in a wheelchair. For twelve years the seventy-two-year-old had been crippled with arthritis in both his knees, his back and his hips. He also suffered from Parkinson's disease. He could walk only with the aid of two sticks, dragging his legs along. I worked on Len for about half an hour, applying my hands to his arthritic joints.

At the end of the session I asked Len if he would like to stand up and test his mobility. Slowly he started to walk, using one stick to support himself and bending his knees for the first time in years. His companion exclaimed: 'I've never seen Uncle Len walk like that before. It's a miracle!' Len seemed not to be able to believe what had happened. He was reluctant to sit down and kept walking around the room, insisting he no longer needed his wheelchair. As if to underline his determination, he walked down the half dozen steps outside the front door and got into his car without assistance.

Fred Ripsher was sixty years old and had been in constant pain since an unsuccessful operation on his spine two years earlier. His mobility was also limited. I began the session, placing my hands gently on his shoulders. After only a few minutes he started to twitch, as though he was receiving a series of electrical shocks, and then shouted, 'The pain has gone!' The medical witness at this session, Dr Christine Pickard, had examined Fred before I began the healing and she now repeated the tests with him. He could lift his arms and legs and bend down to his toes. She said: 'Yes, that's pretty fantastic. The muscles are much slacker.'

Eight of the twelve people I treated as part of the newspaper's experiment reported substantial improvements, which were verified by the doctors. The failures included a paralysed child, a man with a broken leg and a man with thrombosis. The *News of the World* reported Dr Pickard's assessment of the experiment:

All these cases of improvement are compatible with medical teaching – they can be put down to psychological factors. They happened where there was an overlay of muscular and/or emotional tension. Chronic illness always tends to have a large measure of this, because people are frightened. They hold themselves tight as protection against further injury or pain. Their muscles become fixed in a 'unhealthy' position and they become further emotionally upset by the continuing illness.

This was a perfectly reasonable explanation of the state many
of these people had been in before healing, but it did not answer
the fundamental question of how the medical profession had
achieved no result when I had managed to overcome these 'psychological factors' in a matter of minutes.

Timing is said to be everything with some endeavours. So far
as that first British tour was concerned, ours was disastrous. The
summer of 1981 in Britain was a sizzler in terms of social unrest,
which affected my tour. On 5 July the Liverpool suburb of
Toxteth became a 'no-go' area when a mob forced the police to
retreat. I was due to give a demonstration on 9 July at St George's
Hall in the centre of Liverpool. We arrived at the hall to find it
ringed by police, who were expecting further trouble. Word must
have got round because I ended up with an audience of twenty.
The following day violence erupted again, in Liverpool,
Manchester, Birmingham and a number of other towns and cities
across the country.

The evening of the 10th was another big date, at Manchester's
Belle Vue. We got there to find that it had been fire-bombed. We
moved on, to Nottingham, then to Leicester. In Leicester I was
scheduled to give a healing demonstration and lecture in a hotel
called the Grand, where I had also booked a room for the night.
The place was buzzing when I arrived to check in, with hordes
of young girls hanging around the main entrance. I took this as
an encouraging sign, although surmising that they must be
waiting for the owner of the powder-blue Rolls Royce parked
outside. I wondered who that could be.

Later that afternoon a couple of men with very long hair came
in to where I was setting up for my evening presentation. The
leader of their band wanted to meet me, they said. The leader
turned out to be Ritchie Blackmore, who had been lead guitarist
in the recently disbanded super-group, Deep Purple. Blackmore
was apparently in Leicester to play a gig that night with his new
band, Rainbow. I had been a Deep Purple fan since my school
days. Ritchie was proposing that he come to the first half of my

lecture before playing his gig and that we meet at the hotel afterwards. I was not a little in awe of meeting this archetypal rock
figure, and not a little wary. Quite apart from his status as a brilliant musician, Ritchie had a fearsome reputation for volatility.

That evening he was very genial and plied me with questions
about psychic phenomena. Performing had obviously left him
on a high and I stayed up talking to him until late into the night.
The evening I spent with him and his band took my mind off the
disappointing numbers that had turned out for my demonstration.
Wherever we went, the story was the same. The perception of
the streets as unsafe frightened many people into staying indoors.

Life seemed to regain its normal equilibrium during the last
third of the tour. We hoped this would be reflected in increased
attendances. However, only relatively small numbers of people
seemed willing to include me in the process of getting on with
their lives. By the end of the last demonstration, in Southampton,
Graham and I were facing losses running into thousands of
pounds. I had undoubtedly misjudged my pulling power, and
my audience.

Many of the people who were interested in what I was doing
in this country were New Age types. In the early 1980s most of
these people seemed to fit a particular mind-set left over from the
1960s and 1970s. They conformed to what I call the 'poverty
culture' of believing that everything should be free. My demonstrations were not free. Given that venues had to be hired,
programmes printed and accommodation paid for, they could
not be. Everything is a resource and should be valued as such,
whether it is my time and energy or that of the other people
associated with what I do. In my experience people generally
do not value what they do not pay for.

That tour forced me to rethink my strategy of how I was to
establish myself as a healer in Britain. Financially and professionally the States remained my bedrock, and the demand for
my appearances seemed as healthy as ever. The workshops I
gave over here were no different in content from those I gave in
the States and elsewhere. The major difference was in scale.

Overseas I could count on audiences of hundreds at a time, sometimes thousands. In Britain I had to settle for about a dozen gathered in someone's home or in the back room of a pub. In this way I built up a grassroots following and my reputation spread by word of mouth.

My life changed after that tour in one other important respect. I had met my first wife, Christine. When my sister Rosalind introduced us for the first time, I thought she was the most beautiful woman I had ever seen. I found myself repeatedly dropping by the shop where Christine and Rosalind worked. If she had the best pair of eyes I had ever seen, I possessed the best set of wheels she had come across. I have always loved fast cars and at this time I was driving a slinky Lotus Esprit sports car. In our individual ways we turned each other's heads. She was going out with someone else, so I persuaded Rosalind to ask her if she would accept a date with me. Within a few months we decided to live together at Charity Farm, a house I had bought in October 1981.

Since parting company with Win and Charles in 1980 I had done no one-to-one healing. I was spending an increasing amount of my time in Britain making and organizing recordings of healing techniques. I was helped in this by my brother, Andrew, who had worked for a record company. He knew of a state-of-the art and professionally run recording studio near my home in Withersfield, which he said would be an ideal place to record the boxed double tape I was planning to do as a follow up to *Healing and Self-healing* and *Creative Visualization*. This studio was at Claret Hall, just outside the village of Clare in Suffolk.

The double tape I wanted to record at Claret Hall – *Fighting Back* – was specifically about self-healing, and included relaxation, visualization, positive attitudes and, on side four, a relaxation and self-healing exercise. The idea for *Fighting Back* had come out of work I had done with cancer patients, both in this country and abroad. The cancer sufferers I had encountered fell broadly into three groupings of equal size: the first seemed to want an instant response and were not interested in doing anything for themselves; the second were marginally interested, in that they would sometimes make efforts themselves; the third group comprised people who were intent on fighting their disease on several fronts and who regarded healing as only one avenue of help.

While I was recording the main healing meditation, Robert John Godfrey, composer for the band The Enid, who also rented the studio and with whom I had become acquainted, said to me, 'It would sound much better, you know, if you put some music on it.' He volunteered to provide some, using his training as a classical musician.

What Robert came up with was tremendous. Sweeping, emotional, uplifting and empowering, the music for *Fighting Back* was totally different from anything else in the field, which tended to be very short of inspiring. Even now a lot of so called New Age music sounds to me as though it has been produced by someone who has lost one arm and the three fingers of his remaining hand in an industrial accident. He adds a bit of birdsong to the two notes he can play on his portable synthesizer and calls the end result music for meditation or music for healing. After *Fighting Back*, music would become an integral part of my healing practice.

Robert's capacity for alcohol was as astonishing as his musical talent. Many of our sessions for *Fighting Back* were done at night and when we had finished we would go to Robert's 'local', a pub run by an ex-Flying Squad officer who kept the freest house in my experience. He never stopped serving drinks and out of hours would simply close the door and carry on supplying rounds to his regulars, sometimes until five in the morning. It was a drinker's paradise and much frequented by the constant stream of musicians recording at Claret Hall.

Robert's favourite drink was port, and his devotion to it showed in his twenty-stone frame. On our first outing together I was memorably introduced to this wonderful wine and unwisely helped him consume a bottle and a half. I was so ill, I thought I was going to die, or at the very least suffer severe blood poisoning. That should have been a warning, but instead of being put off port, I developed a taste for it.

Robert and I became regular drinking partners, either at the pub or at Charity Farm. He and the other Enid band members, Steve Stewart and Chris North, would sometimes come over to us for dinner. We would get into enormously long discussions and ferocious arguments during which time simply evaporated. On more than one occasion we sat around the dinner table from eight in the evening until the milk was delivered at seven the next morning.

Whenever I got the opportunity to publicize what I was doing, I took it. In January 1982 I was invited by Anglia Television to appear in a programme called *The Healers*. It was a very straightforward 'trial' of various therapies. I was presented with two people and asked to give them both healing. The first person, a publishing executive with a painful knee, did not benefit from my treatment. The second person was a woman with an infection of the hip joint. According to her doctor, who was interviewed on the programme, the only way of controlling her condition was with painkilling drugs.

At the end of about twenty minutes of healing the woman (who insisted on remaining anonymous) said that the pain – which had been with her constantly for two years – had gone. A year later, the pain had still not returned. The woman, who professed to being completely sceptical about 'faith healing', said: 'It can't happen – but it has!'

I have a Methodist Minister, Reg Watson, to thank for becoming accepted by Christine's parents, both of whom are very devout Christians. They were uneasily aware of my healing. Early on in my relationship with Christine, Reg gave a talk at the church attended by Christine's parents in which he told of his experience of healing. He had had cancer of the prostate gland and pelvis for about a year before coming to me. His doctors had given him a few months, possibly weeks, to live. I do not know what Reg said in that talk, but the following is his description of his illness and his experience of healing:

I got to such a point in my life where I was literally dying by inches. I lost two stone. I had tremendous pain, such pain as was beyond all my human imagination, like somebody holding a blow-torch against my pelvis and buttocks. My left leg was paralysed almost totally to the big toe.

The medical treatment left Reg:

...numb from my belly button to my big toe, but it didn't kill any pain. It numbed the muscles but didn't do anything for the nerve. The first day Matthew gave me treatment, after about five seconds I knew something tremendous was taking place, in my body. My response was phenomenally powerful, and the experience has strengthened my faith in God. The first day I knew I was going to be healed. I simply knew it was going to happen.

Six months later, with regular healing and the use of creative visualization techniques, Reg had regained the two stone he had lost.

I had a favourite expression which I still use dozens of times a day as a kind of prayer. I ask God to use the laser beam of his healing power to destroy the cancerous cells and I can see them being bombarded and absolutely destroyed. And they are being, that's the marvel. . . . I don't suppose I've ever been happier in my life than I am right now.

Reg's story helped Christine's parents to lose any lingering suspicions they might have about me or the spiritual correctness of healing.

In April 1982 Christine and I got married quietly at Cambridge Registry Office. Neither of us wanted a Church wedding with all the attendant fuss. The only people present other than the Registrar were my brother and my secretary, who acted as witnesses. Christine and I decided that we would dress down for the occasion instead of up. When the Registrar came out to greet us, he mistook my secretary and my brother for the bride and groom, and thought Christine and I were two scruffs plucked from the street outside to stand as witnesses.

Shortly after our marriage I decided to rent an office above a butcher's shop in Bury St Edmunds. I needed a base from where I could run the tapes business, which seemed to be taking on its own momentum and growing faster than I had anticipated, or indeed wanted. The response to *Fighting Back* had, however, encouraged me to produce more tapes to help people with specific health problems, such as allergies, insomnia, depression and osteoarthritis.

The philosophy behind the tapes was simple – heal thyself. This was not a new idea but the enormous possibilities it offered seemed lost on those who should be embracing it. I had made *Fighting Back* to show people how to use positive methods to overcome problems, and to encourage those sporadic self-helpers to do more for themselves. The tapes were a way of reaching a wider audience. The reaction to *Fighting Back* was very encouraging, with orders coming in from doctors and local health centres, as well as from private individuals who had picked up the tape in health stores.

Gill Hurd of Loughborough personified the attitude I was trying to impress upon the people seeking my help. She had first come to me in 1979 when I was practising from Charles and Win's premises in Leicestershire. Some years previously she had had a mastectomy, from which she had fully recovered and 'led a totally ordinary life and never thought about cancer', until she was shown X-rays of the disease in her lungs.

Gill believed that her cancer had been caused by an accumulation of stress: her husband's business had not been doing well, she had started a new job and a close friend had died. Life seemed to be made up of a series of bad happenings.

Her husband, Bill, was told that her condition was incurable and that she had only three months to live. Gill 'knew the situation was pretty bad', and was determined to do something to help herself. As well as taking the drug prescribed for her, she made big changes in her lifestyle, including revising her diet, taking exercise and using my healing tape, *Fighting Back*. Then she began to see me regularly for healing. She reported: 'When it got to Christmas I felt very emotional because I had not expected to live that long. Although I was very positive, deep down I did wonder whether it was going to be my last Christmas. I wanted to get all the family round. I felt as if it was probably the last one.'

After that first period of intensive healing, Gill came to me about once a year. This is how she saw the healing process she was experiencing:

> **I think Matthew is a very strong channel of healing energy. Sometimes I feel great heat; not always. I feel very much better after one of our sessions and that feeling lasts for days afterwards. I always feel it's a recharging of the batteries, and I go away inspired to continue with all my efforts.**

Fourteen months after the initial diagnosis the hospital asked Gill to have a scan. When she went back to get the result from her consultant, he looked at her, at her notes, at the scan and then back again at her. She sensed something was not adding up for him. Eventually he said: 'Well, I've got your scan results. I've got good news and bad news for you. Which would you like first?'

Having spent over a year working on herself positively, Gill opted to hear the good news first. 'The good news is we've got your scan results back. We've scanned every part of you – your lungs, your liver, your bones and your brain – and you are completely clear. We can't see any trace of the cancer anywhere. I don't know what you've done, but, you can ask your husband, I told him last year that I thought you only had three months to live.'

Having been given this news, Gill said 'That's fantastic, isn't it? But if that's the good news, what's the bad news?'

'The bad news,' he said, drawing in a very deep breath, 'is

that you must live with the knowledge that, unfortunately, it will eventually come back again.'

Incensed by his negativity, Gill did something that was quite out of character. She got out of her seat, banged her fists down hard on his desk, and shouted, 'The hell it will!' That became the motivating factor in keeping her going. She was determined to prove him wrong, and it was the springboard from which she launched a cancer self-help group in her area. She has told me:

> I felt all along that there was some strong purpose behind it all ... I think I've been the catalyst in bringing together the people that helped me ... At the time I felt very over-privileged that so many people wanted to help me. I thought, 'What have I done to deserve all these people helping me?' I felt I must give something back.
>
> My whole attitude has changed. It sounds a very strange thing to say, but having cancer has taught me so much that I wouldn't have missed the experience.

Ironically, after Gill set up her cancer support group, the consultant who had so angered her sent many of his patients to her. Hopefully, his eyes were opened to the possibility of there being more to getting better than receiving conventional medical treatment.

Gill said to me many times that she was determined to die of something else to prove him wrong. The cancer did, in fact, return and she died in September 1997. Whether she would have had those eighteen additional years of life without receiving healing is anyone's guess. Her spirit and attitude made them rewarding for others as well as herself. Gill embodies my belief in how healing, in its fullest sense, can spread from its source and benefit other lives.

Another of my patients was a lady who suffered from multiple allergies. As well as receiving healing, she doggedly followed my suggestions for self-help, meditating for five minutes three times a day. She confirmed what I tried to impress upon patients without making the regime seem too onerous:

> You have to do the work and have to do it regularly. It is
> not a magic wand you wave.... Initially I was feeling quite
> ill, with a lot of pain all over and becoming quite crippled.
> I was losing the use of my fingers and my hands were
> drooping ... I can drive again, I don't get depressed. I can
> eat – that is the biggest thing – I can eat! My own doctor
> just cannot believe the difference in me. He was giving
> me strong painkillers, five lots a day, just so I could get
> some sleep. Now I don't need them.

In practical terms the recording side of my healing enterprise was threatening to take over my life. Part of the problem lay in my streak of perfectionism. Whatever I undertake, I want to do it to the utmost of my ability. Many New Age products seemed to lack quality. I wanted all my tapes to be attractively packaged and up to the standard expected by the wider public. A great deal of effort and money had to be invested in them to ensure that they were.

The only aspect of the business I liked was making the tapes and deciding how they should look. I had no interest in the practical side of making a return on what had been expended. I just expected it to happen. At the end of 1982 I decided that the best plan would be to employ someone else to handle sales to enable me to concentrate on healing.

In early 1983 I started to use the premises in Bury as a healing centre, to accommodate the increasing number of people wanting to receive one-to-one treatment. The philosophy I projected in my workshops and demonstrations, and in the tapes, underpinned the principles of the practice. Anyone who came to me, I decided, must be prepared to work at mental and physical exercises to help their illness. This was spelled out to people enquiring about treatment – and put quite a number of them off!

Many illnesses are, I believe, stress-based, and it is sensible to insist that people try to tackle the problems causing their stress. Often simple techniques such as deep breathing and relaxation will alleviate the situation, but these have to be taken seriously and integrated into the person's lifestyle.

My patients in those early days had to get used to my insistence on them taking responsibility for their illness. The attitude of many doctors then discouraged people from taking an intelligent interest or asking awkward questions about the treatment being proposed.

In September 1983, Sheila Lawler of south London was diagnosed with cancer of the cervix. She undertook a course of radiation therapy, which seemed to have a beneficial effect. A short time later it was discovered that the cancer had spread to the lining of her bladder. Her doctors suggested radical surgery, involving a colostomy and removal of her bladder and other parts. Sheila was waiting for a hospital appointment when a friend showed her an article about me.

After our first session Sheila told me about the course of treatment her doctors were suggesting. I gave my usual non-committal response: the decision had to be hers. 'That annoyed me,' Sheila said later. 'Instead of advising me, my guru was telling me to make up my own mind. Yet Matthew must have sown a seed because after the healing I felt so well, so confident, that I began questioning the surgeon about the operation and analysing his answers.'

Sheila was told the operation would be long and difficult, but it would give her between five and ten more years of life. Without the operation, she could expect to have between eighteen months and two years. The quality of her life, however, would be better, because the operation would leave her facing many problems and indignities.

'I decided not to have it and once I'd made up my mind, I felt really elated. I believe Matthew gave me the strength for that decision. I'd been on a strict diet, but that night I celebrated with a fish and chip supper.'

Sheila is still alive and well at the time of writing and has had no hospital treatment since receiving healing.

✳   ✳   ✳

On 11 October 1984, Henrietta was born. Her arrival confirmed what marriage had already suggested – that it was time for me to cut down on touring abroad. Christine had often travelled with me, but with our new baby making three, this was no longer possible and our existence became more settled and centred on home. Overseas tours were no longer as financially necessary either. The number of people coming to see me at the centre was gradually increasing and I was confident that this would continue.

There is no more influential medium for getting one's name and face known than television. Three years after *The Healers* for Anglia came a proposal for a half-hour-long documentary from BBC Television East. This promised to treat what I was doing seriously and to draw on the positive evidence for the efficacy of healing provided by interviews with some of my patients. It was just the kind of exposure I needed.

When the film was eventually viewed by producer Mike Purton's superiors, it was rejected for being 'too pro-Matthew Manning', and a further day's filming was insisted upon to redress the perceived imbalance. I suspect that many television executives regard controversy as being synonymous with interesting viewing. The counter-balancing the studio bosses had in mind consisted of trying to make something out of the fact that I charge for treatment. Was it ethical to make people pay for a gift given by God? I argued that the talent of a footballer, an artist or a musician is no less God-given than my own, yet no one questions their right to earn a living from it. I try to be fair and have devised a system that ensures that those who can afford to pay for treatment are supporting those who cannot.

The most rewarding aspect of the film was hearing the stories of the patients selected for interview. One of these was told by Dan Hutchison, a fifty-five-year-old retired tax consultant with an interest in alternative medicine. He had been diagnosed with a rare form of cancer. He had a tumour the size of a small melon in his right adrenal gland and the cancer had also spread to his liver. He had lost six stone in weight, felt constantly tired and was by his own admission 'in a very low state indeed'.

Dan told me: 'Statistics showed that nobody with this form of cancer had survived. They said I would require an operation, and on being pressed they admitted the chances of a successful operation were about one in a hundred. Without the operation they told me I could only put my affairs in order and look forward to about six months.' Dan declined the operation. I felt, and Dan agreed, that he was so weak that he would initially need intensive treatment. He came twice a day every day for a week. Dan said: 'After each visit I felt in a very relaxed state. Even after the first visit upon leaving his room I reached the car and discovered I was carrying the stick. I had needed that stick up until then.'

After a few months Dan's brother, who was a doctor, found Dan 'in a remarkably good state, so much so that he suggested that we go out for a walk, and we walked and we walked, and we discovered that we'd done about five miles over the Chiltern Hills. I felt wonderful.'

There is an encouraging postscript to Dan's story. In 1992, eight years after he had first come to me, he got an unexpected letter from the hospital that had first diagnosed his cancer, the John Radcliffe Infirmary in Oxford, offering him the opportunity of having an MRI scan. (MRI stands for Magnetic Resonance Imaging, which has replaced X-rays in the detection of malignant tumours and other disorders.) Dan's name had come up on their computer records and they were obviously surprised that he was still alive. His wife had been badgering him for years to go back to the hospital and have a scan, but he had always resisted, fearing that he would worry if the tumour was shown to still be there.

Dan did go back and the MRI scan showed that the tumour had completely disappeared. The only trace of its existence was some scar tissue. (Dan died of a massive stroke in 2003.)

The documentary was shown in the BBC TV East region in late 1985 and created such a response in viewers that it was screened nationally on BBC2 in spring 1986. Ironically, at this precise time my fortunes had dipped to their lowest point. Passing on the management of the sales side of the tapes business turned out to be anything but a smart move. The people I had hired were incompetent, and still expected to be paid handsomely. By the end of 1985 the debts from that business had forced the sale of Charity Farm and left us with the princely sum of £1,500.

Chapter 5

DARK NIGHTS OF THE SOUL

I was totally unprepared for the avalanche of interest generated by the television documentary. Our telephone lines were jammed with calls for days afterwards and I received thousands of letters, each one of which had to be answered individually. When the film was screened nationally about four months later, in early 1986, I was better able to deal with the response.

One of the benefits of this exposure was that it finally imprinted on people's minds my identity as a healer. Several people were confused by my evolution from teenage psychic, believing that my father had been the centre of the poltergeist activity and that I had taken up healing independently. Explaining was a small price to pay for the shift of consciousness I had been trying so hard to bring about. The 'Poltergeist Boy' image was happily laid to rest by the media, too, now that they had an exciting 'new' label for me, and they began reporting on my healing work with refreshing seriousness.

Previously, I had been waiting for word about my healing work to spread gradually by personal recommendation. Now there were not enough hours in the day to cope with all the demands on my time. I was determined to make the most of this change in fortune. Personally Christine and I were going through a miserable time. We were now living in a tiny terrace cottage situated in a village called Woolpit, near Bury St Edmunds, where Christine had no friends and no means of regular escape because she could not drive. My having to be away from home so much did not ease her sense of isolation, but we were in a catch-22 situation – either I worked all hours to get us out of the place or I worked less and we stayed there longer. I elected to work all hours.

The appointments diary at my healing centre in Bury was permanently full and invitations to give workshops were coming in from all over the country. These were largely confined to weekends and evenings, with the occasional two- or four-day event.

The numbers attending the workshops had been creeping up before the programme, from around fifteen to over forty. Now I was regularly attracting over 100 people per session, and sometimes as many as 250 in the larger centres. I had got used to seeing the same groups of 'regulars' around the country. I like to get to know my audiences, to scan their faces as I talk, and develop a rapport. I had to familiarize myself with the influx of newcomers. Some of them were undoubtedly trying me out, as they would a new product or fashion item, and were probably not genuinely interested in healing.

When the unmistakable features of comedian Jasper Carrott leapt out at me during one workshop in London, I thought – after convincing myself that it was indeed him – that he must be gathering material for his shows. He seemed earnest enough, though, exchanging energies with other people and taking part in the other exercises. At the end of the session he asked me to sign a book for him. He told me that an interest in dowsing had led him into healing. When I teased him with my initial suspicion, he said I did a far better job of sending up healing than he ever could!

A year later Jasper sent me tickets for a show he was doing in Ipswich. To my amazement the first story he told was a variation on one I had used in that workshop, about an area around where I live which is known locally as the Suffolk Bermuda Triangle because every time you get to a certain point the signs direct you back to where you have just come from. Jasper's sole attempt at a disguise was to change the place-names to those around his native Birmingham.

By the mid-Eighties the belief that man must change his wasteful and destructive ways to ensure the continued survival of the planet was being taken far more seriously than previously. One of the organizations responsible for helping this process was the Wrekin Trust, an educational body set up in 1971 by New Age pioneer Sir George Trevelyan with the aim of '[awakening] the vision of the spiritual nature of man and the universe'.

The Trust ran many events throughout the year 'to help people develop themselves as vehicles for channelling spiritual energies into society'. Its most prestigious event was an annual conference, 'Mystics and Scientists', which gathered together Christians and Buddhists, humanists and sceptics, to discuss the ideas that continue to separate materialists from non-materialists.

I felt tremendously pleased when the Trust asked me to present a workshop under its auspices. One of the exercises we did during that workshop was an old favourite I had been using for years, involving the left and right sides of the brain. Most of us are dominated by the left hemisphere, the rational, analytical side of ourselves, which overshadows the creative, imaginative us. Rarely are we aware of what is going on in that right side because we are too busy rushing around or being anxious about some aspect of our lives. We need to be deeply relaxed or have our senses heightened to get in step with it. The point of the exercise is to show how the two sides can be enabled to communicate to achieve inner balance and harmony.

Workshops attract many different types of people, and I have often wondered what each person takes away from the experience. I like receiving feedback from people so I can assess what they are getting out of what we are doing together. There is always room for improvement and I am constantly looking at ways to present material more effectively. Some people become very chatty and open once the initial shyness barriers have been lowered. Others are more self-contained. I try to let everyone find their own level of comfort within the situation while making the atmosphere as relaxed and informal as possible.

One man at the Wrekin Trust workshop was unusually quiet, never asking any questions and keeping himself very much to himself. He would turn up each morning sweating profusely, as if he had come a long distance, with a bicycle clip clinging tenaciously to one of his legs. At the end of the workshop I discovered that he was the singer-songwriter Van Morrison. I was not a particular fan of his work until I heard *Poetic Champions Compose*, which was released some months later and became one of my favourite albums. Its appeal lies in what it gives back to me in understanding. I do not know whether some of the ideas expressed in it were inspired by that workshop. I thought so when I heard it for the first time, especially the track 'Did you get healed?', and in 'I forgot that love existed' there are two wonderful lines that encapsulate what I was trying to get across in that left/right brain exercise –

> *If my heart could do my thinking*
> *And my head begin to feel*

The focus of my workshops is always the people themselves and showing them how to develop their own abilities. I try to keep myself out of it as much as possible, using the healing demonstration at the end merely as an aspiration and proof of what can be achieved. Many people are amazed by what the exercises teach them about themselves and the hitherto unsuspected perceptions they possess.

Joyce Owen came to one of my workshops for no reason other than that she was acting as chauffeur for her husband, Tom, driving him down to London from their home in the north of England. She stayed only to appease her husband, but insisted on sitting near the exit so that she could escape at the earliest opportunity. Joyce had been a nurse and her interest was caught by the exercises, which were designed to identify the causes of illness, to be aware of other people's problems and use techniques such as guided imagery to control pain and bring about self-healing.

When I asked for a volunteer for the demonstration at the end, Joyce was the most suitable candidate, having restricted movement in her neck which, if the healing worked, could be shown to be improved. Joyce told us that her consultant had admitted that he could do nothing more for the osteoarthritis in her neck and that she would have to spend the rest of her life wearing a surgical collar. She could not take painkillers because of a peptic ulcer which the medication she had been given to control the arthritis had caused, and manipulation of the neck was, according to the consultant, too dangerous to be contemplated.

Joyce sat down in the chair I pulled up for her and made herself comfortable. She demonstrated how far round she could turn her head. On the left side, this was hardly at all. I asked Joyce to think about something she enjoyed doing while she listened to the music I was about to play.

At the end of the session, I asked Joyce if she had felt anything. She responded: 'Yes, I felt terrific heat going through my neck from side to side and then from back to front. It felt like a ball of heat about as big as a tennis ball. Although it was very hot, it was not at all uncomfortable.'

'Were you aware of anything else?'
'Well, yes. I felt you gently moving my head up and down.'

I was very puzzled by this, because she had kept her head absolutely still, and I had not attempted to move her head. Indeed I had not touched her neck. The only touch had come at the outset, when I had placed my hands on her shoulders for a couple of minutes. The rest of the group, including her husband, assured Joyce that there had been no manipulation. I asked Joyce to demonstrate how far she could move her head now. The right side was unaffected by the arthritis and so moved normally, as it had before. The change in the left side was startling. She could turn her head without stiffness, creaking or pain. I was as delighted as Joyce. Now that her neck was unlocked, I told her to try to keep it that way, by gently exercising it regularly.

Joyce went away and followed my advice, but after a few months her neck was again painful and aching, although the movement was not restricted. Unconnected with this development, Tom expressed a wish to visit the Healing Arts Exhibition in London. Neither of them knew that I would be there, too. I spied Joyce as she was buying one of my tapes, *Relief from Pain*, and went over to her for a chat. She told me that her neck seemed to be trying to 'lock up' again.

I was not surprised her neck muscles were grumbling, given the number of years they had not been used properly. I offered to have another 'go' at them and began to give her healing on a regular basis. Seven years later her neck was still permanently pain-free, and fully mobile. She continued to have healing for the arthritis threatening other areas of her body – for her knees, in one of which the cartilages were shown, by arthroscopy, to be almost completely destroyed, and her hips. These show marked improvement, and she can now run upstairs, climb hills and play golf.

So much of what I do has evolved through trial and error, and leaps of imagination. The healing circles that made up such a large part of my work in the Nineties were a good example. The idea to connect energy came about as a spontaneous response to a particular situation.

During a demonstration in Birmingham, I had asked if anyone present had a hearing loss; this is a good ailment to demonstrate in public, because any improvement in it after healing will be obvious to the rest of the audience. Seven hands rose in the air, far more than I had anticipated. It made more sense to give them all the benefits of healing than to waste time conducting a hearing test. The only way I could imagine doing this was by inviting the seven on to the stage, standing them in a line, getting them to hold hands, and giving healing to the person at what I designated the head of the row. I asked the other six to imagine the healing as electricity running down a wire.

At the end of this demonstration the hearing of the man on whom I had placed my hands was vastly improved, as was the hearing of everyone else in the line. Subsequently I used this idea of connecting energies during my workshops – although this threw up another problem.

Sometimes the healing would reach a certain person in the line and no further. In some instances I suspected that the energy was being deliberately 'blocked', probably because the person responsible was more interested in trying to cut me down to their size than using their energy positively. This was very unfair to the other people in the group. I soon figured that the way of circumnavigating all future 'blockers' would be to place people in a circle. With this configuration only the 'blocker' would suffer.

* * *

In any other sort of business the unrelenting workload I was piling on myself would inevitably have led to stress. I was fortunate in that my work provided the tools for keeping me in a stress-free zone. During those perpetual tours of the States I had used a lot of Silva Mind Control techniques to hone my creative visualization skills. Meditation, a crucial skill for a healer, had come very naturally. I virtually taught myself, by experimenting and talking to people who were experienced meditators. Once I began to heal professionally, I found I could switch into a meditative state almost at will. There are limits, however. I discovered mine on the day I met the actor John Cleese.

Cleese's assistant called with a request for an appointment on that very day. Cleese was in urgent need of attention after aggravating an old injury to his knee while filming one of his manic runs. We had one slot left for later that afternoon and as none of the people waiting on our cancellations list had a more pressing claim on my time, it was decided to give him the appointment.

On being asked for instructions on how to get to Bury St Edmunds from London, we told the assistant that Cleese could either drive or take the train. He opted for the train, which runs from Liverpool Street station, as do most services from London to Essex and the East Anglia region of the country.

Unbeknown to us until later in the day, Liverpool Street had been where Cleese had aggravated his knee, while shooting the opening scene of the film *Clockwise*. In the film he plays a head-master who has been invited to give a speech at a headmasters' conference in Norwich. He arrives at the station, approaches a railway official and asks if that is the train to Norwich, pointing in the direction of one of the platforms. He interprets the mumbled reply as 'Yes' and gets on the train.

The conference is a very important event for him because he will be the sole representative from a comprehensive school. He gets out his notes to begin revising his speech and is soon lost in a reverie of applause and admiration. After a while he looks at his watch, then out of the window, and suddenly realizes he is on the wrong train and that the right train is moving out from the next platform. In panic he leaps off the stationary train and runs – in exaggerated Basil Fawlty style – along the platform after the departing train. It is while he is catching his breath from this failed attempt that he notices the train he was on moving out of the station, taking his speech notes to he knows not where. The rest of film is about what befalls him as he tries to reach Norwich in time to give his speech.

Cleese himself must have had a curious feeling of déjà vu at some point after his arrival at Liverpool Street station to catch the train to Bury St Edmunds. He bought a ticket, quizzed a railway official about the whereabouts of the train, misconstrued the reply, boarded the wrong train and only realized his mistake after the right train had departed for his destination. We received a call from his assistant to say that he was on his way, by black cab, but that he would be late. He eventually arrived at the end of the day, and related his extraordinary tale. His amazement at what had happened was capped when the cabbie who agreed to drive him from London to Bury St Edmunds asked if he was going up there to see me.

Giving treatment to John Cleese was about as problematic as his journey. He is enormous, like a telegraph pole. The only way I could effectively reach his knee was by having him stretched out in a chair while I sat cross-legged on a cushion on the floor with my hand on the affected part. It is not easy to forget who John Cleese is when he is in front of you. Merely his face makes me want to laugh. He does not have to do or say anything.

As I put on the music at the start of our session, I told myself that I must not look at him. I sat down on the cushion and began to concentrate. After about ten minutes I thought I could hear him sniggering. I chided myself for being fanciful and told myself he was probably engaging in deep breathing. The impression of sniggering kept coming back to me, though, and after a while the sound of laughter was unmistakable. It became progressively louder until he was bellowing so loudly I should think anyone passing in the street outside could hear him. My concentration now completely broken, I opened my eyes and looked up to see Basil Fawlty laughing manically. I must have looked worried. He said: 'Don't worry about me. This is how I get rid of my stress.'

At the end of the session he settled his bill and made a large donation, which he asked me to use for people who could not afford to pay for healing. Cleese had not thought to ask the London cabbie to wait for the return journey, so he was forced to risk the homeward journey by train. The least I could do was take him to the station, although I wondered how he and a bumper bag of nappies for Henrietta were going to fit into my small Renault. As we started walking to the car, he said, 'Give me the nappies. If I'm carrying them, people won't think I'm John Cleese.' He strode along, ignoring the turning heads and wondering looks. Sure enough, no one could believe that John Cleese would be abroad during the rush hour in Bury St Edmunds, swinging a bag of nappies.

The healing did not solve the problem with his knee. The fact that it did not was disappointing. However, it was not a life or death matter. Sometimes it is.

We live in a culture that seems to find it increasingly difficult to interpret or cope with the grey areas of life. As we 'progress' so the expectation grows that all ills can be cured by one means or another, and if they cannot be the outcome is termed 'failure'. My first 'failure' had taught me not to get carried away with the idea that I could make healing work every time. That power is simply not in my gift. It has not always been easy telling people that I cannot be sure how the healing will go. Illness is a strange phenomenon, however, which seems to bring out an understanding of life – and death – that probably resides in most of us. The more healing I give the more sure I am that its purpose goes beyond the physical. People seem intuitively to open up to the idea of healing working on levels that they might not consider in the normal run of daily life. There is a touchstone of certainty about the purpose of our lives that crops up time and again in the letters and messages I receive.

Nicola Waller was only fifteen when she first came for treatment for cancer, at Easter 1984. Healing was a last resort of her parents, who had been told she probably had no more than a few weeks to live. She was brought for healing regularly and I also taught her to use visualization techniques to fight her illness, by imagining her body destroying the cancer cells. Her mother, Jean, said of Nicola's treatment:

> She gained another eighteen months of normal living. She had her treatment, and like everyone else in the hospital she was made extremely ill by the chemotherapy. Each time I would bring her to see Matthew and she just bounced back. It changed her attitude. She had a greater appreciation of life. She enjoyed life. I know personally what she gained, how she gained. She knew that she was going to die. There was no fear. She was very, very peaceful. Very happy. He never promised to heal the body. He said it could have been the mind that he healed. And in this case I am positive that is what happened.

Each act of healing also seems to have its own dynamic in relation to the people supporting the patient. In the case of Patrick Sheehan the emotional repair work effected by healing extended to his daughter, Bernadette. Patrick had been told by doctors that he had only two weeks to live. At this point Bernadette wrote and asked me to give him healing. In the six months of life that were, in fact, given to him, he underwent a transformation that enabled Bernadette to, in her words, 'love [him] again unconditionally. I saw him in a totally different light. He became again the father he once was, and one I thought I had lost forever.'

*   *   *

The response I was getting directly, both at the workshops and in one-to-one sessions, indicated how far the circle was widening, drawing in more and more people. If numbers and enthusiasm are any guide, there was an almost palpable opening of minds to the possibilities inherent in healing. I felt sure it would be only a matter of time before the medical profession acknowledged the potential of healing, and other hitherto 'suspect' therapies, and embraced it.

I saw orthodox science and orthodox medicine as a couple of curate's eggs – good in parts. However, I had met enough highly intelligent, open-minded doctors not to think those good parts of the orthodox medical egg were miniscule. I understood, too, from my conversations with Kit Pedlar and other 'renegades' how the negative attitude towards non-orthodox methods of treatment had come about. Years of brainwashing had gone into instilling that hostility, with trainee doctors being warned against 'quack' therapies.

As doctors were no longer being trained to be prejudiced, there seemed a good chance of a significant number among present and future intakes being able to look at complementary therapies objectively. One of the people responsible for re-inforcing this optimism was Brian Roet, who had been introduced to me by LBC Radio's phone-in doctor, Michael van Straten. Several of my patients had asked me if I could recommend a hypnotherapist. I did not know of any and so I asked Michael,

who put me on to Brian. His questioning spirit has led him on
from his original training as a general medical practitioner into
anaesthetics through to hypnotherapy and latterly counselling.
Brian exemplifies the ideal of medicine as an ongoing process in
which practitioners are constantly searching for new ways of
helping the process of healing.

As he would write in his introduction to *Matthew Manning's
Guide to Self-healing*:

> The more we learn about ourselves and our self-healing
> potential, the less likely we are to require drugs or
> 'someone else to fix us' by injections, operations or the
> multitude of laboratory tests now 'routine' in the medical
> profession. I hope one day the work of healers like
> Matthew will be alongside the medical profession –
> acknowledged, understood and a part of the healing
> routine available to those in need.

Thinking can be contagious, or so it seemed to me in 1986 when
the Royal Society for Medicine asked me to be one of a quartet
of speakers to address its oncology section on the topic of complementary therapies in the treatment of cancer. I decided
beforehand that this had to be an occasion for winning friends
and influencing people if the 'complementary' ideal was to take
root in the minds of my audience.

Complementarity not competition was the unspoken theme
of that speech. I stressed the need for multiple approaches in
the treatment of cancer, of there being no single omnipotent
branch of the healing arts which had all the answers. I was
not seeking to replace conventional medicine or advocating
that it should be allowed to wither on the vine. I wanted to
feed the notion of partnership – between the scientific and
technological innovations which enable improvements in diag-
nostic and surgical techniques, and therapies which provide
nourishment at all levels to allow patients to retain a sense of
themselves and of their importance in the treatment equation.

I outlined the aspects of healing which I knew from experience were important to people and were increasingly perceived to be lacking in conventional treatments – touch, communication, understanding, empathy. These were the elements the medical profession should be trying to integrate into its way of working. Complementary therapies provided the means. I did not add that the medical profession could learn a great deal from its nurses who, because of the hands-on nature of their work and closer relationship with the people in their care, seemed to be more comfortable with these elements.

The other speakers invited to address the Royal Society for Medicine that evening were Dr Rob Buckman, Dr Patrick Pietroni and Dr Jacqueline Filshie, all of whom had trained conventionally and were now using complementary therapies.

Buckman, a cancer specialist who had emigrated to Canada in 1985 after being frustrated in his aim of establishing a training scheme for junior doctors, was well known to British TV viewers as co-presenter, with Dr Miriam Stoppard, of *Where There's Life* and *The Buckman Treatment*. In 1978 he had contracted a life-threatening degenerative disease, dermatomyositis, in which the body's auto-immune system attacks muscle, and had succeeded in overcoming it with the help of a battery of different disciplines, including 'alternative' techniques. Jacqueline Filshie was a highly respected anaesthetist who was pioneering the use of acupuncture in surgical operations as an alternative to anaesthetics.

The remaining speaker, the 'alternative' general practitioner Dr Patrick Pietroni, wanted to see the widespread introduction of complementary therapies into orthodox medicine. For some reason he got the worst reception of us all. I suppose there was no point in them trying to shred Buckman. He was no longer part of the British medical scene, and beyond their reach. All they could do was sit and grind their teeth quietly while he extolled the virtues of the Canadian system with its very different approach to cancer medicine and comparatively lavish resourcing. Pietroni, by comparison, was in the throes of establishing a National Health Service general practice with

complementary practitioners on site at his Marylebone Health
Centre in London. He was a true pioneer. Ten years later nearly
40 per cent of general practices in Britain would be offering some
form of complementary therapy.

That evening seemed at the very least to signal a willingness
on the part of some in the medical establishment to take stock of
their traditional attitude of wholesale hostility towards non-
orthodox forms of treatment. The two sides were like ageing
feuding relatives who were at last willing to acknowledge each
other's good points. However, although the psychological log-jam
was clearing and the lines of communication were now ostensibly open, there were still pockets of resistance, ready to snipe
when the opportunity arose.

A few years after that evening at the Royal Society for
Medicine, I was invited to give a one-day workshop to a group
of health-care professionals from the oncology departments of
two hospitals. The principal topics I covered in that workshop
were healing, self-help, relaxation and positive attitudes. The
venue was Keele University, and the audience was composed of
doctors, nurses, counsellors and several cancer patients. The
medics organizing the event were sympathetic to my work, but
not all of their colleagues were as open-minded. One of the
organizers warned me about a highly sceptical consultant in the
audience. I asked the doctor to point him out. I do not like confrontation, but I do like a challenge.

When it was time for me to demonstrate healing, I invited the
consultant to select somebody for me to treat. I said it might be
helpful if he were to examine the person both before and after the
healing, so that he could give the audience the benefit of his observations. He introduced one of his patients, who had undergone a
mastectomy and radiotherapy for breast cancer. He explained that
several muscles had been cut during surgery and that a nerve in
her shoulder had been damaged by the radiotherapy treatment. As
a consequence of these injuries, she was in considerable pain and
her ability to move her arm was limited. He very much doubted
that healing would bring about any improvement.

The consultant went back to his seat and I began to work on the lady in question. Fifteen minutes later she was moving her arm in all directions for the first time in months and declaring that all the pain had gone. When I asked the consultant if he would like to re-examine his patient, he got up and shouted 'I'm not getting involved in this circus', and stormed out of the hall. I am not sure what he meant by this, unless he believed – as many sceptics do – that people feel under pressure to 'perform' when they are in front of an audience and that the benefit they say they have derived from the healing is purely psychological. I have no way of knowing whether the improvement that woman experienced was sustained. If the consultant had been prepared to discuss the case, it might have been possible to establish some form of monitoring.

The consultant's use of the word 'circus', however, suggests that he might have been confusing healing with some of the woollier organizations clustering around the fringes of the 'alternative' movement. Credibility in the wider world largely relies on perception, and the fact that there are some very vague practices masquerading as therapies or carriers of enlightenment has hindered the cause of the genuine. Graham Wilson, the promoter of the Festival of Mind, Body and Spirit, has always tried to promote the proven end of the range of complementary therapies on offer each year. Part of the publicity campaign to attract ordinary people through the turnstiles has involved asking Festival participants with a relatively high public profile to 'plug' the event.

Whenever the media has requested names to interview, mine has tended to be among those put forward. By the late Eighties, it seemed that some people in the media were getting bored with playing the Festival straight. The political correctness of taking us seriously was wearing off – for television, at least. One year they decided to confront perceived whackiness with intentional whackiness in the form of Ruby Wax. I would have quite relished the chance to spike her guns, but it was not to be. She refused to deal with me, because, she told me, she had too much respect for what I was doing. Instead she had sport with the veteran colour therapist Theo Gimbel, who, overwhelmed by this unexpected opportunity, was flummoxed into confirming that the wearing of red underpants provided effective protection against AIDS!

I hasten to add that I am sure colour therapy has therapeutic, though limited, value in some cases, and that it can contribute to an overall feeling of well-being; it is not by accident that my healing room is papered in a particular shade of yellow. As with any therapy the question of what it can genuinely offer to the patient has to be addressed. I can think of no possible circum-stances in which the claims of some of the organizations sheltering under the 'alternative' umbrella can be taken seriously.

I shall never forget trying to sort out the confusion sown by the reassuringly sane sounding Aetherius Society. The name makes me think of enlightened learning in wood-panelled sur-roundings, a sort of British Library for those who split their time between earth and the astral plane. In fact, it was the brain-child of a London cab driver called George King (later Sir, after his self-elevation to the peerage), who established the group in 1956 after allegedly hearing a voice which told him to prepare himself 'to become the voice of Inter-planetary Parliament', apparently a body of spiritually advanced beings living on other planets which is keeping a kindly eye on us earthlings from a fleet of UFOs moored somewhere in the galaxy.

Two people who had been exposed to King's ideas found their way to my stand at the Festival one year. In this early period of the Festival's life, I used to take a stand as well as give demon-strations, workshops and lectures. Over the five days people would come up for a chat or just to browse through my stock of cassettes, books and videos on healing. I did not pay much atten-tion to the two men in question until one of them stopped, looked at what was on offer and sidled up to me. Rather self-consciously, he said, 'I wonder if you could give me some advice.'

I said, 'Sure. Tell me what the problem is and I'll see what I can do.'

'Well, it is of a rather personal nature. Would you mind if we just moved over here because I don't want anyone else to hear what it is?'

When we were out of earshot of anybody else, he said, 'Actually, the problem is not mine. It's my friend's. He's got rather a big one.'

I was unsure whether to keep a straight face or fall about laughing. I opted for the former and, rather foolishly, asked, 'How big is it?'

'Well, it goes out about ten miles.'

Realizing now that we could not possibly be on the same wavelength, I probed a little further and discovered that his friend's 'problem' had been discovered during a visit to the stand of the Aetherius Society: two adepts had 'dowsed' around him and proclaimed him to have a ten-mile aura. Perplexed by this startling piece of information, the two men had set out to overcome what they took to be a problem of matching proportions. They had managed to solve half the problem, and were hoping I would be able to take care of the other half. I was intrigued to know how.

The man said, 'We've bought a seafront flat in Brighton, and so long as my friend stays in the flat, half his aura is going out across the sea, although he does occasionally get shipping going through it. We wonder if you've got any advice as to what he can do with the other half, because it's got a bus terminal in it, a very large road and the city centre.'

I could not believe that anybody could be so completely serious about something so utterly nonsensical. I am still not sure whether one of the men was raving mad, whether they both were or whether they were just two gullible souls who believed everything they were told. Out of mischief, and also for want of knowing where else to send them, I advised the man to take his friend round to the stand of the National Federation of Spiritual Healers. It did not seem appropriate to offer him healing. Indeed, I will not give healing if I feel there is no likelihood of it doing some good. This is the sole principle that guides my decision of whether or not to give healing.

In the mid-Eighties I found myself being challenged by a vociferous minority to deny help to AIDS and HIV sufferers. The vindictive controversy whipped up by the media was undoubtedly fed by fear. The tabloids especially were enthusiastically publishing stories about the 'gay plague', and peppering them with quotes from moralizers who saw the disease as Divine retribution for promiscuous and degenerate living.

When it became known that I was giving healing to a number of people infected with the virus, I was bombarded with letters – most of them from born-again Christians and members of fundamentalist Christian Churches – which expressed horror that I should be prepared to help such 'outcasts'. I was not prepared to play God and bow to the pressure applied by these people. I hit back as hard as I could, and tried to shame them into seeing how un-Christian their attitudes were.

The hostility that HIV/AIDS provoked in the general population is now, thankfully, a memory, but in the mid-Eighties it was as large a component in treatment as the virus itself. As in cases of cancer, the aim is to strengthen the immune system by adopting relaxation and visualization techniques and changing negative fears into positive beliefs. Combating the virus effectively involves removing the stresses that conspire to weaken it. I can think of no more demoralizing stress than being made into a pariah.

One of my patients – a man – confided: 'People stand up in the pulpit and denounce you, shun you; they do not want to know. They do not want to help. There are very few willing hands to hold yours.' At that time the stigma attached to the virus could overtake the effort to fight it, and suicide was often uppermost in the minds of people when they discovered they were carriers.

With the support of his wife, that man did not act on his initial impulse to hang himself and eventually succeeded in overcoming his shock and fear. 'Everything we had ever dreamed of suddenly went down the chute. No children. No nothing. Everything vanished and we suddenly had just this one goal.' He came to believe in his own powers of healing and redefined his approach to life. 'I think peace of mind will definitely prevent an occurrence. I have every chance of surviving and I cannot see any reason for not surviving. . . . I am not under stress. I am perfectly calm and nothing is going to worry me.'

*　　*　　*

The doctor who introduced me at the Royal Society for Medicine told his audience: 'People are voting with their feet, and we have to find out what it is that people like Matthew Manning are offering them.' In some cases I think this could be summed up in one word, 'hope'.

Eberhard Fuchs and Barbara Steinsch were among the several foreign journalists who asked for interviews after the broadcast of the documentary on me. They came to Britain and spent the best part of a weekend with Christine and myself, talking about healing and selecting case histories that they could follow up. The material they gathered was originally intended to run for six weeks in a German mass-circulation women's magazine, but such was the response from readers that a further five articles were commissioned.

Shortly before these articles were published, I had received a letter from the mother of a little girl called Anja Kowalska, who was then two and a half years old. Her mother, Eva, wrote that she had been born three months prematurely, weighing just two pounds. A week later she had suffered paralysis of the part of the brain that controls movement, and the ability to sit, stand, speak and focus the eyes. On three occasions during her first week of life, Anja was declared clinically dead. The doctor treating her at the Munich Paediatric Centre had put the chances of her making a slight recovery as low as 1 per cent and had told the Kowalskis that she would never be able to raise her head, let alone speak or walk.

Anja was in a wheelchair when I first saw her, a lifeless bundle that could have been mistaken for a floppy rag doll. I impressed upon Eva and her husband, Heinrich, that I could make no promises. I had no experience of this sort of case and so could not predict whether healing would have the result they were seeking. I could only try.

During our three healing sessions Anja would perspire so heavily that her clothes had to be changed. I interpreted this as a sign that some process was underway which would shortly yield results, although Anja's condition showed no improvement. I advised the Kowalskis to return with Anja in a few months' time. Eva confided to me later that she had gone away bitterly disappointed.

Exactly two months after the first visit, Anja's eyes began to improve markedly – so much so, in fact, that a planned operation was cancelled. The squint was still there, but the eye specialist was confident that it would 'sort itself out'. Anja then tried to raise her head, and a few days later she looked at her mother and smiled. Eva was overjoyed to receive this first expression of Anja's love. She could barely believe her ears when a few moments later, the child suddenly said, 'Mama'. 'Papa' and 'Doro', the name of her older sister, were the next words.

A month later the Kowalskis flew back to Britain with Anja. After another three healing sessions, she was refusing to wear a nappy and demanding a potty! She could now sit up on her own and speak complete sentences in German and in the Kowalskis native tongue, Polish. Soft-boiled egg and white bread became her favourite foods. Slices of sausage she could eat on her own. Anja showed further improvement during a third visit. The morning after the first healing session of this trip, Anja took her first steps, holding her mother's hand. A few months later she could show her mother how a bird flies, moving her arms like wings.

The consultant treating Anja could offer no explanation for the change in her condition. Convinced that the improvement in Anja was due to my healing, the Kowalskis were desperate to continue bringing her to see me at regular intervals. However, their finances were straining to meet the cost of air fares and accommodation. I rang Eberhard Fuchs to assess the chances of a German magazine being interested in sponsoring the family, perhaps in return for the right to publish Anja's story. Eberhard succeeded in securing a deal with *Frau Aktuell*, who asked the Kowalskis to provide an ongoing update on Anja's progress. Anja's case was widely reported in Germany and the Kowalskis received many letters from desperate parents wanting to contact me.

*   *   *

For Christine and me, March 1986 to March 1987 had been our first annus horribilis. The only good thing about it was that it came to an end, and at that end I had earned enough money to enable us to move from Woolpit. Our choice was a medieval house in one of the main streets of Bury St Edmunds. Its main attractions were the attractive disused mill that it overlooked at the back, and its convenience. I could walk to work and Christine would not feel my frequent absences so acutely in a bustling town environment. We would both be happier.

1987 also marked the end of my love affair with the United States. I had been back only once since 1984, for a week in 1986 to give lectures and workshops. In 1987 I did this again. Both trips were organized by Denise Linn, before her evolution into a teacher of personal growth. In the early Eighties I had considered the idea of moving there permanently and even gone so far as to apply for a Green Card. It seemed to make sense when I was working there for three months solidly and only seeing home for a few days at a stretch between tours. In those years I must have covered virtually every town in America, other than the Bible Belt and the Southern states.

When I did go back I saw how the scene had changed to become just another facet of corporate America. A lot of the fun and naivety had gone out of it, and the 'gurus' themselves were jostling for commercial advantage in what was becoming an overcrowded marketplace. The most successful 'gurus' were those prepared to promise instant results, whether it was enlightenment, weight loss or contact with celestial beings. That had never been my route and I was not about to tread it. The States was no longer the place for me.

This no longer mattered now that I had built a large following in Britain. Professionally I could get along very comfortably without having to cross the Atlantic. I kept working as hard as I could, fearful that if I did not I might lose everything again. When I was at home with Christine we would relax in the company of the new circle of friends we were making in and around Bury St Edmunds. Heavy drinking was becoming a way of life for both of us. Away from home it eased the loneliness, if only for a night. When I was out socially with Christine, it made me feel just like the next man. The people with whom I came into contact through my work tended to elevate me, despite my efforts to make them believe in their own abilities. Perhaps this is a natural reaction: only if we believe someone is better than us do we take any notice of them or their message.

I did not want to spend my spare time being deified. The people I came across socially reacted in one of two ways to the fact of my being a healer. Either they would make a caustic comment before picking up their drink and moving to the furthest corner of the pub, or it would become the sole topic of conversation. A comfortable point between being the centre of attention and being cold-shouldered was sometimes difficult to find. I did not want to tell people what I did for a living for fear of their reaction. I figured that if I drank as much as the rest of them, there could be no question of me being regarded as different.

In private Christine was certainly doing her best to tell me I was not special. The negative comments which had started when we were living in Woolpit took on a sharper edge. Problems had arisen on the few occasions she had accompanied me on tours before Henrietta's birth. People had tended to ignore her and on some occasions had been downright rude. Understandably, this treatment had upset her and caused rows between us. Now that she was staying at home while I travelled alone, she suspected me of making the most of her absence. With me or not, she felt excluded. Rather than find ways to ease the situation, I looked for opportunities to be away from home and out of earshot.

*　*　*

The interest provoked in Germany by Anja Kowalska's case encouraged *Frau Aktuell* to invite me to give two lecture/healing demonstrations in September 1988, one in Hamburg and the other in Bochum. I was in two minds about accepting the offer. Germany had become one of my least favourite countries. On the other hand, I do not like turning down invitations, especially ones prompted by public interest. I decided that if the magazine was prepared to risk of incurring the wrath of petty officialdom, so was I. The authorities might take a different view of my activities this time, because of the enormous publicity that cases such as Anja's was generating.

Hamburg lived up to its reputation as a city-state that has always gone its own way, trading and thinking as it pleases. I had a full house of people wanting to hear what I had to say and eager to see the healing demonstration. There was no obvious official presence, no threatening watch on my activities. Immensely relieved, we moved on to Bochum, an unremarkable town in Germany's industrial heartland.

All was going according to schedule until a few hours before I was due to appear on stage. A telex message was received in the offices of *Frau Aktuell* from a Dr Martin Segerling, who described himself as having overall responsibility for the health authorities in and around Bochum. In his message Dr Segerling stated that the practice of healing was illegal and that, although I was at liberty to lecture, I was not permitted to demonstrate healing. After hurried consultations with one of its lawyers, the magazine decided that Segerling's threat should be ignored and that I should go ahead and give both the lecture and the demonstration.

About twenty minutes before the start of the lecture, four uniformed policemen arrived at the venue and demanded access for themselves and a small group of people accompanying them; under German law none of them could be refused entry. Dr Segerling, we learned, was among the party of accompanying officials. Another member of his plain-clothes brigade approached me and asked if I was Matthew Manning. As soon as I confirmed that I was, he thrust a sheet of paper into my hand. This turned out to be the German equivalent of a High Court injunction ordering me not to demonstrate healing.

The magazine had taken the precaution of sending its lawyer, Herr Haendeler, in case of trouble. I asked him what would happen if I ignored the injunction. The police had the power to arrest me the instant I laid so much as a finger on anybody, he said. I would then be taken away for questioning, and probably be fined the equivalent of about £200. This did not seem too bad, and I mulled over the idea of being a martyr until he pointed out that having a criminal charge against my name would make it very difficult for me to get back into Germany.

Reluctantly, I decided that I would have to comply with German law. It was frustrating to be in the same situation as the last time I had visited the country, but there was no sensible way around it. My spirits were raised considerably when it became clear that Herr Haendeler was intent on discomfiting Dr Segerling and injecting drama worthy of press coverage. He was not the lawyer of a mass-circulation magazine by accident. Haendeler asked me to give my talk and then hand the meeting over to him.

At the end of my lecture I explained to the audience that I was being prevented from giving the advertised demonstration of healing. As expressions of anger rippled around the packed hall, Haendeler joined me on the platform. He announced that *Frau Aktuell* would refund the full cost of every ticket. Then he read out the text of the court order served on me. When he had finished, he challenged Dr Segerling to come on stage and explain his action. This was a neat move, because the by now loudly simmering audience needed to vent their disappointment on someone and fairness demanded that it should be neither me nor Haendeler. Segerling could not be heard for several minutes above the chorus of abuse and taunts accompanied by loud stamping.

The uproar proved too much for one elderly gentleman, who collapsed. I could not believe my eyes when not one of the doctors in Segerling's group was moved to help him and his care was left to other members of the audience. Eventually Segerling made himself heard above the din. He confirmed that no healing was to take place, and that if it was attempted the full force of the law would be used to stop it. He stuck doggedly to his point: that he was maintaining the law. The burghers of Bochum did not thank him for his rectitude and booed him off the stage.

After Segerling's hurried departure, I addressed the audience again, apologizing for what had happened and offering to come down among them to answer any questions. The stage seemed unusually high and I felt more comfortable talking to people informally at ground level. I left the stage and was soon surrounded by dozens of people in the hall, some wanting advice, others wanting to express their outrage at what had happened. I do not speak German and was concentrating hard on providing my answers to the many questions in simple English. In the background I became aware of Eberhard's voice, shouting, 'For God's sake, don't shake hands with anybody!' I looked up to see the four uniformed police officers standing on chairs, staring into the throng of people, waiting for me to touch somebody.

The next morning the German press had a field day and gave the event in Bochum far more coverage than would have been the case if I had been allowed to give the healing demonstration. I drew no comfort from this. In blocking me the authorities had also succeeded in preventing some of their citizens from receiving help. It is this aspect of the opposition to healing which has always caused me most sorrow and anger.

✳   ✳   ✳

After years of being accepted more readily in other countries than in Britain, where many people seemed not to know what to make of me or what I was doing, the pendulum now seemed to be swinging the other way – with obstacles abroad and recognition at home. Some of the people who were coming were persuaded by the experience of close friends, as in the case of Robin, Marquess of Tavistock. He had suffered a massive stroke in February 1988, which he survived against all the odds. He was discharged from hospital about two months later, still weak from his ordeal and with a range of disabilities to overcome. In addition to being slightly paralysed on his right side and blind in his left eye, he had severe speech and memory problems. When he first came to see me, his speech was improving and vision was beginning to return to his left eye.

According to the Marchioness, her husband did not believe in healing but was encouraged to come to me after I had helped a friend of his, antiques dealer John Partridge, to regain his sight. She said:

> I went along with him and sat in the room while Matthew put his hand on my husband's head. He immediately felt warmth. And the really strange thing was that I could actually feel it too.
>
> After the first visit my husband looked incredibly peaceful, was very happy and said that he felt so much better. After further sessions he regained 80 per cent of his vision in his left eye, which was the one that had been badly affected by the stroke, and his dysphasis – which is being unable to find the word you want – has improved immensely. He now believes.

Sarah Fletcher also came to me in 1988 on the advice of a friend. She was told she had a cancer rating of three after receiving a positive result in a cervical smear test conducted at the John Radcliffe Hospital in Oxford. The laser treatment proposed then had to be postponed when Sarah discovered she was pregnant because of the danger it would pose to the unborn child. A friend suggested that she try healing to counter the worsening in her condition that was likely to occur before the conventional treatment could be given. Sarah said of her first visit to me: 'He placed his hands near me, not quite touching my body. Afterwards, I felt extremely relaxed and very hot. It was as though I'd experienced some sort of heat treatment.' She came for another session two months later. In January 1989, her baby, Melissa, was born. Two weeks later Sarah had another smear test. The result was negative.

Nicky Bilton's problem was also gynaecological and causing her, in her own words, 'excruciating pain':

> I was told that the only way the problem could be definitely diagnosed would be to have my womb removed and the tissues analysed.
>
> By the time I decided to go and see Matthew, I had stopped work and was living in a fuzzy world, on prescribed painkillers and gin, which is a uterine relaxant. The first treatment was quite amazing. The feeling of heat was so intense that it was like being burned alive from the inside and the searing sort of pain that accompanied it was an enormous relief. Then after each session, I just felt more and more relief. After six months I went back to work and after a year the pain had gone.

*　*　*

I am convinced that the people who need my help will receive it, because somehow our paths will be made to cross. In May 1989 I was giving a workshop in Totnes, Devon, when I was

approached by a woman who asked me if I would see her two-
and-a-half-year-old daughter, whom I shall call Charlotte. The
case was very unusual, and the paediatricians at the local hospital
had referred Charlotte to Great Ormond Street Hospital in
London for a diagnosis. I explained that I would be happy to
see her once the condition had been diagnosed. A few weeks
later, I received a letter:

> Great Ormond St Hospital did lots of tests but cannot
> make a definite diagnosis although they seem convinced,
> because of the [CT] scan, that it is a rare leucodystrophy
> [a progressive degenerative brain disease]. The only
> further diagnostic test is a brain biopsy. As they are sure
> it is untreatable, it would be heartless to put her through
> that ordeal.
>
> Now I am tearing my hair out, trying to find the person
> who can help to cure her, and all the NHS seem to want
> to do is provide pushchairs, places in special schools,
> counselling and attendance allowance.
>
> [Charlotte's] posture is now failing; she sits with her
> back bent and her head down looking at her navel. I'm
> afraid her left hand is becoming clumsier; she asks to be
> helped with feeding although she can just do it on her
> own. Her intellect is still perfectly normal and her spirit
> is amazingly buoyant for someone who can hardly do
> anything on her own.
>
> . . . If you think you can help the sooner the better as
> she deteriorates daily in spite of our prayers and deter-
> mination.

Charlotte was clearly an urgent case and I saw to it that she was
given an early appointment. She had three sessions of healing
over a period of six months. In a letter to me, her mother said:

> The first time we came I was stricken with fear and agony
> at her deteriorating state. She could barely eat or speak,
> although she was sitting much more positively. Within

three days she started speaking audibly and asked to get out of her pushchair and push. She has never looked back, going from strength to strength.

Of Charlotte's final session with me, her mother wrote: '. . . When she got out of the car and ran in and chattered away I was so happy and couldn't stop grinning. I could see straight away that she'd had another boost.'

After her final visit Charlotte was taken back to Great Ormond Street for more tests, including another CT scan. The first scan had shown degeneration in white matter on both sides of the brain and 'unexplained 'tissue' between the hemispheres of the brain'. The abnormality in the white matter was still apparent in the second scan, which Charlotte's mother described as

> . . . a dark symmetrical area on both sides with a rim of white when it should all be white. I was so dumbfounded at there being no obvious change that I couldn't ask them to elucidate. Of course they are perplexed and mystified too . . . All they can do is make informed guesses based on previous experience and they say [Charlotte] is unique. They think it could be an unusual reaction to an infection, but this usually shows up as patchy areas of abnormality. They didn't think anything I had done was a radical breakthrough, although they did not by any means dismiss the fact that a positive attitude, faith and determination are powerful forces.
>
> . . . I wish I could understand it all and come to some conclusion, but there isn't one and there are many. I decided I had to know for better or worse what had happened in her brain, but now that I know it's the same, I don't know what to do with that knowledge. I'll have to just accept it as a fact.

Charlotte's return to good health has continued, as her mother confirmed in a letter she sent several years after the healing sessions:

She is a flourishing seven-year-old now, enjoying school
life, and has no memory of there ever being anything
wrong with her. She still can't ride a bicycle and I think
her balance and coordination are slightly impaired but
on the other hand I couldn't ride a bike or swim until I
was eight and she can swim! She reads and writes
extremely well and, although we were a bit worried
when she first started school, she makes slow but steady
progress and compares favourably with her peers.

Charlotte's story demonstrates that there are no limits to the
power of healing. A feature of leucodystrophy is the disruption
– in some cases destruction – of the means by which electrical
impulses are conducted through the nervous system, thus dis-
abling the system and preventing it from performing its functions.
Charlotte's doctors came to the conclusion that somehow the
electrical signals were being rerouted through another part of
her brain. Quite how this has been achieved, they are at a loss
to explain. More important than the 'how' is what cases like
Charlotte's teach us, as her mother confirmed:

> It really has been the most awesome experience anyone
> is likely to have. I always thought we were lucky not to
> have her snatched from us abruptly, and that it was such
> a joy to be able to have her and be happy with her living
> life for the moment for however short a time, but to have
> her restored to good health clinically, if not technically, is
> miraculous. Anything is possible.
>
> The greatest thing I have learned is the power of love
> and positive thought.

Elisabeth and Hans Büscher displayed similar determination to
Charlotte's parents in exploring every avenue to help their sick
child, Vanessa. In September 1990 the couple brought her to see
me from their home on the small island of Fehmarn, off the Baltic
coast. Lack of oxygen around the time of her birth had resulted

in Vanessa being brain-damaged. Despite a gloomy prognosis, the Büschers left no therapeutic stone unturned in their attempts to improve Vanessa's situation. When swimming, gymnastics and perception therapy failed, they turned to healing. One healer in Munich promised them a cure.

They made the 700-kilometre journey to the south of Germany twelve times in a period of three years with no perceptible improvement in Vanessa's condition. Shortly afterwards Vanessa began to show signs of severe disturbance, raging, screaming and beating herself for hours at a time. The Büschers were recommended to try a magnetizer in Holland who told them that he would be able to relieve her distress but not her disability. After three weeks of treatment, Vanessa was noticeably calmer. At around this time the Büschers read about Anja's case, and made an appointment for her to see me. Elisabeth wrote of that first visit in a letter sent to me in August 1992:

> Vanessa was then eight years old, dainty, small and looking at most like a five year old. She could walk, when held with both hands. On stairs she had to be carried. Mentally she registered little and still beat herself. My impression during the first consultation was that Vanessa was moved by you and your music and even loved to be touched by you. I hardly recognized Vanessa and was amazed by how calmly she enjoyed your touch.

I told the Büschers that I felt something would change within the following three months. My experience of this type of case had taught me that an instantaneous improvement was highly unlikely. Elisabeth confirmed this later:

> ... after a short time Vanessa became much more awake and alert. At the end of November, this was also confirmed by Vanessa's school.... On the 8th January 1991 began a completely new phase: Vanessa was able to walk unaided! At the time of writing this letter it is still a mechanical walk but she is gaining in confidence.

For further treatment we were again with you in April and November 1991, as well as in April 1992. Vanessa has in the meantime continued to make progress. She can now climb the stairs to our flat alone. On the down climb she still needs our assistance. She can eat on her own and drink out of a cup. Vanessa goes on her own to the toilet!

Language wise, however, little has changed. Sometimes we get the feeling that at any moment words will pour from her like water out of a fountain, but they remain only indistinguishable sounds.

. . . Never would we have imagined it possible that Vanessa could ever walk on her own, and the doctors cannot believe that this is the same child they treated three years ago!'

In cases like Anja and Vanessa's, healing seems to have boosted them from a state of severe handicap to a plateau somewhere short of complete recovery. In such brain-damaged children the effect of healing seems to diminish after the age of eleven or twelve, probably because the cerebral circuitry gradually loses its plasticity and ability to adapt. All concerned have to accept that further progress is unlikely, and be thankful for what has been achieved.

* * *

I had always intended my practice in Bury St Edmunds to be more than just a place from where I would give hands-on healing. My workshops and talks were about self-development and the part healing plays in it. I wanted people to be aware of the many other equally valid disciplines that might help them to achieve wholeness. I launched a magazine, *Attitudes*, which I hoped might fill in some of the gaps in their knowledge and understanding. Under one roof we were running a healing practice, a magazine, a recording business and an informal advice centre. I became accustomed to people popping in to see me to shake hands or talk or get advice.

The place seemed to become a magnet for dowsers. The major ley line in Britain runs from St Michael's Mount in Cornwall – which, ironically, is close to where I was born – to the abbey ruins in Bury St Edmunds. The dowsers who sought me out were intrigued that my centre should be on the end of the line and wanted to know if my energies were helped because of this. I could not confirm that they were significantly. The places where I gave demonstrations were not, so far as I was aware, noted energy hot-spots, and the results of my healing there seemed no less successful than those I was getting in Bury St Edmunds.

Although I was amenable to people coming into the centre informally, there were limits to my hospitality. I am not a particularly proprietorial person, but I do need a space in which I can relax and be unavailable. My bolt-hole at the centre was my office. When I was in the treatment room or the public area in the centre, I would give my time and attention fully. When I was in my office, I was available only to colleagues and friends. One afternoon, though, my space was invaded in the most irritating manner imaginable.

I found a hippy type with a ponytail half-way down his back sitting in my chair with his feet up on my desk. I was so taken aback by his effrontery that I let him start talking. He told me his name was Walter and that he had been dowsing the ley line. He explained that he had wanted to meet me since reading the Norwegian writer Erik Dammann's book *Beyond Time and Space*, which viewed healing within the framework of quantum physics. Dammann's ideas had caused a shift in thinking about healing, and Walter calculated that now would be a good time to publish my recent book, *Matthew Manning's Guide to Self-healing*, in a Norwegian edition, and proposed himself as the publisher.

Despite now being gently warmed by Walter's charm, I hesitated. It is odd how in certain circumstances or states of mind we recycle disparate negative episodes. My experience of hippies in business had been costly, and my suspicions made me wary. Walter had to spend months talking me round and showing me how organized he was before I relented. A few months before

the scheduled publication date, he asked me if I would promote
the book in Norway. Again I hesitated. This time I was panicked
by the thought of what staying with him would entail. He had
proposed that I be his house-guest in order to keep down costs.
I was all for that, but not for the diet of mung beans and spring
water that Walter's appearance seemed to promise. As it turned
out, I was worrying unnecessarily. Walter's appetite for mung
beans turned out to be no larger than my own.

My reception in Norway far exceeded my expectations, and
bore out Walter's belief that there was a large audience for
healing as I was presenting it. In general healing had a bad name
in Norway, partly because of the conservatism of the establishment and partly because of the rather weird approach taken by
Norwegian healers, whose rituals had served to limit its interest.
Many people thought healing was not for them because they
could not relate to the mystical flummery in which it was usually
shrouded.

My style of healing seemed to connect at a very deep level in
Norway. The numbers I attracted to the lectures and healing
demonstrations I gave on that first visit were astonishing, given
Norway's population of about four million (one million of them
in the capital, Oslo), which is some fourteen times smaller than
that of Britain. On my second trip I filled the 600 seats of one of
the largest indoor halls in Oslo.

One of the first healing demonstrations I gave in Norway was
to Elsa Nordhagen, who had recently had an operation on her
lower back that had left her in great pain. She had been driven
to the workshop by her husband, spending the entire journey
lying on the back seat of the car. Elsa also had a frozen shoulder
and, unbeknown to me at the time of the healing demonstration, several tumours in her abdomen.

After the healing Elsa could move her arms freely and the
pain in her back was much better. She told me that she was
supposed to be in hospital that day being operated on, but had
insisted upon the operation being rescheduled when she discovered that it clashed with my workshop. She had booked for

the workshop months before the hospital appointment came through and had been determined not to miss it. The hospital had obliged and she was now due to have her operation a few weeks later.

When we parted, I said jokingly, 'Make sure they scan you before the operation.' She went for a scan on the day after the workshop. On this occasion her doctor confirmed that the tumours were still there, though the largest of them was much reduced from its original seven centimetres. When Elsa went into hospital for the actual operation, she made herself very unpopular by insisting upon having another scan. The doctor could not believe his eyes when the scan failed to show any tumours. Bemused, he asked a colleague to conduct another scan. This scan also revealed no trace of the tumours, and Elsa was sent home without being operated on. Her pelvis and shoulders have not given her trouble since the healing either.

It was lucky for Elsa that the workshop and the date for surgery were separated by three weeks. In her case this was sufficient time for the process started by the healing to produce a result. Elsa's experience also confirms that it is not necessary for me to place my hands directly on the area of the body affected by a health problem. At the time of treating her, I was not even aware of the precise nature of her problem, so this too is not a prerequisite for the healing to do its work. The energy seems to find areas of weakness or imbalance and work on them regardless.

Thanks to Walter's efforts, Sweden and Finland opened up to me after Norway. When I was not working in Britain, I was journeying between venues in these countries. I was inundated with requests to give healing on a one-to-one basis. I was already using the principle of healing circles in my workshops to meet an expressed need among all the participants to experience healing for themselves, and not just get a report of what it was like from someone on whom I had chosen to demonstrate.

When I also began receiving requests to show people how they could send out healing to people they knew, it seemed a good idea to develop an exercise in which everybody could join but which would incorporate the additional boost of my 'battery'. Walter and I therefore started to organize healing circles, adding a new dimension to my work.

In the circles it became apparent how central the emotions are to the efficacy of healing. Physical problems are less likely to occur if the emotions are in balance. In my experience, healing the body necessitates sorting out the emotions first.

Lillian Takvam Nagell was a lawyer working for the Norwegian Department of Justice before a severe whiplash injury caused by a car accident confined her to bed for several months. Her movement was further restricted by rheumatoid arthritis. By the time she read about me, she had already tried a range of treatments to improve her condition, none of which had had much effect.

Lillian enrolled for one of my workshops and, during a healing circle on the second day, experienced a tremendous reaction. In her words, 'Matthew Manning went around the circle and touched everybody for a short while. When he touched me, a very strong wave of energy washed through me, and I felt a deep peace and gratitude. I had had no expectations, so I was quite bewildered about my reaction.'

Lillian's husband collected her after the workshop and they started the long drive to their home. Lillian cried for almost three hours during that journey, releasing long-buried memories of her mother, who had died of a brain tumour when Lillian was eighteen. Afterwards, she told me, she felt very much at peace. During the three days after the workshop she was able to step out of herself and see her life from a distance, recognizing previously undiscovered patterns and connections.

When Lillian woke up on the third day, she was free of pain for the first time in several years and felt a tremendous joy of life. She could move in such a way that the injured area between her shoulders was more relaxed and her circulation was greatly improved. The most important aspect of the transformation she underwent at this time was the evaporation of fear, especially of death. Lillian said she had previously been one of those people who is afraid of everything – of the dark, of flying, of illness. For the first time in her life she felt safe and enveloped by love.

The extraordinary feelings Lillian experienced gradually subsided in the following weeks and months. Initially this return to normality distressed her and she wondered what she had done wrong. Then she realized that she had to be the one to take herself forward and tackle the life that was waiting there for her. The healing had been the tools, but the means lay in her own heart and mind:

> One of the most important things Matthew says is that you must have the willingness to confront yourself. To me this is about taking hold of the things you have suppressed and stored away. It can be a tough process sometimes. I can see I have only just started this work, but what has been of great help to me is that I have learned how important forgiveness is and to have trust in the process of life.

* * *

Two opportunities to return to Australia presented themselves in the latter half of 1990. Graham Wilson's Festival of Mind, Body and Spirit had expanded to include Sydney and as a regular I was invited to take part. A couple of months before the Festival, in August, I gave a series of workshops in Sydney and Melbourne with flautist Tim Wheater.

Tim's career in music was delightfully eclectic and included jazz, classical and rock. Initially a student of James Galway at the Eastman School of Music in New York, he had then entered the world of pop, playing with Roxy Music, Bronski Beat and Eurythmics. His transformation into a New Age composer and performer had been instigated by serious illness, from which he had recovered with the help of natural therapies and the power of music. His debut solo album, *Awakenings*, had been written

as a stress antidote and like much of his music is dreamy and
uplifting.

When I first met Tim he was studying the role of music in
psychology and, in effect, looking at ways of creating sounds
that were both therapeutic and musically interesting. A great deal
of our material dove-tailed and we started to give combined
workshops, taking it in turns to share personal experiences and
demonstrate practical exercises. At the end of the workshop we
would arrange everyone in a circle and Tim would play while I
went around giving healing.

Even away from his flute, Tim was a pied piper, so we had a
lot in common. This was just as well because we were sharing a
beach-side apartment in the Sydney suburb of Manley. On our
last night there, we were invited to a party by a mutual friend,
Stuart Wilde, who had been enormously successful in the States
at putting across his ideas on personal empowerment and
positive thinking. He had written several books and lectured
widely; *The Answer to Money Is Having Some* is one of his titles.
As well as being honest and intelligent, Stuart was entertainingly
over-the-top and theatrical. I liked and respected him immensely.

I had only drunk a bottle and a half of wine by the time we
arrived at Stuart's wonderful home overlooking Sydney harbour.
No sooner were we through the door than he started preparing
a special drink, placing a bottle in a saucepan of water and
lighting the hob. I had not drunk Saki before and so the ritual of
heating it to body temperature before drinking it was new to
me. I was also ignorant of the fact that it is a kind of Schnapps,
and drunk in very small measures. Stuart filled a large wine glass
and handed it to me. I did not think twice when he told me to
throw it back in one go. That is my last recollection of Stuart's
party. I stayed on my feet for about thirty seconds before crashing
to the floor. I was out cold until the following morning.

When I came round, I was violently sick and felt terrible. The
one thought in my head was that somehow I must make the
flight home. I regained consciousness around noon, which gave
me a couple of hours to get from Stuart's place to the flat in

Manley, pack my belongings, and drive to the airport. When I reached the flat, a fresh-faced Tim told me that Christine had telephoned in the early hours and had reacted angrily when he told her what had happened, suspecting that a woman must be the reason for my absence.

I felt too ill to worry about what Christine was thinking and dragged myself off to the airport. I got there in time, boarded the plane and organized myself, intending to spend the entire journey resting. I could hear fussing and rustling from the seat behind me as an elderly woman eventually succeeded in stowing her plastic raincoat and matching headgear in the overhead locker. We were still on the tarmac when she called the steward to ask him to retrieve the articles she had spent so long putting out of reach – God knows why as we were not likely to be exposed to the elements for hours.

The steward opened the locker and out tumbled a full bottle of duty-free Advocaat onto my unsuspecting head. Still semi-comatose from the effects of the Saki, I was now completely 'out' for the second time in about fourteen hours. I came to after a few seconds, unsure quite what had happened, to a cacophony of screams and expressions of horror. Blood was pouring from a head wound, soaking my shirt front.

The cabin crew insisted that I should be taken back to the terminal to have my head stitched. The last thing I wanted was to take a later flight. I just wanted to get home. After a brief tussle of wills, they agreed to delay the flight while the wound was attended to. The doctor I saw was persuaded to do just enough to staunch the flow of blood, enabling me to get back on the plane without too much delay. In spite of my bloodied state, I was told I had been upgraded to first class – a move probably calculated to reduce the chances of my lodging a formal complaint with the airline. Given the choice, I would have preferred a clean shirt. Fate was wearing its ironical hat that day. In their effort to humour me the cabin staff brought round lists of fine wines. I could not face any of the vintages on offer and slept all the way home.

Christine was waiting for me at Heathrow Airport. She was shocked by my state, but would not believe me when I explained how I had got into it. At that time, Christine was desperate to have another child. We had taken no precautions since Henrietta was born, but try as we might she could not get pregnant. Every month she would be plunged into depression and our already strained relations would become more tense still.

Ironically, I seemed to have no problem getting women pregnant through healing. Anne Farmer had initially come for treatment in spring 1987 after she and her husband, Derek, had been trying unsuccessfully for a baby for about two years:

> . . . I had tests done at the hospital which they said con-
> firmed that my Fallopian tubes were blocked even though
> they could offer no explanation as to why. Before these
> tests I was given a course of Clomid tablets [fertility/-
> hormone drug], but to no avail. You agreed to help us and
> to the surprise of my consultant at the hospital I did
> become pregnant. Unfortunately I lost the baby at eight
> weeks. The fact remained, however, that we had proved
> the hospital wrong – obviously the Fallopian tubes had
> become 'unblocked'. I was prescribed Clomid treatment
> again and with your very special help my husband and I
> succeeded in having a healthy daughter, Lisa, born on 17
> September 1988.

Five months after Lisa's birth, Anne and Derek began to try for a second baby. After fifteen months of disappointment the couple began to feel that history was repeating itself. Her doctor prescribed another course of Clomid. Five months into the six-month course of this treatment, Anne wrote to me again, on 23 May 1990, with a view to coming for healing as soon as possible after the conventional treatment ended:

> If I fail to conceive I have been told I will have to go
> through the same infertility tests as before. They were
> very unpleasant and I am dreading the thought of another

laparoscopy, which is usually standard procedure, especially as I feel I don't really need these tests again. I have
always believed that it was your special help that brought
us our daughter, and if you would be prepared to help us
again this time I would be eternally grateful.

A few months after receiving healing, Anne conceived, and on 3
October 1991 she was delivered of an 8 lb 7 oz boy. He was
named Luke Matthew Derek in recognition of the two 'fathers'
Anne was certain had been involved in his creation.

Elaine Carpenter had tried to get pregnant for two years
before having tests that revealed fibroids the size of melons:

I had these removed but the operation left me with adhe-
sions on both my ovaries.

I stopped ovulating and another fibroid was discovered.
I was told there was very little chance I could become
pregnant unless I had a further operation.

I booked in for the operation, but in the meantime
decided to go and see Matthew. During the first visit, I
felt warm and very peaceful and must have conceived
almost immediately afterwards.

* * *

The place where we were living had turned into a nightmare.
The mill and the plot of several acres on which it stood were
sold off to a property developer, who bulldozed it and erected a
four-storey block of flats on the site. Gone was the pretty aspect
and large expanse of sky. It was like having a black cloud
hanging permanently over our small courtyard garden, casting a
deep, depressing shadow. All the charm went from the place,
leaving me feeling oppressed and desperate to get out. I longed
to find somewhere in the country and eventually stumbled across
it in a village some ten miles south of Bury.

Sturgeon's Hall had fallen on hard times and was in an
advanced state of dilapidation. It was just what I was looking for

and large enough to serve as a home and an office. The lease on
the centre in Bury was nearing its expiry date and it seemed
senseless to search for new premises in the town when pedes-
trianization of the centre was hampering the efforts of many of
my disabled patients to reach me for treatment. From my perspective it was the right time to be moving out. Christine came
reluctantly, saying she was unhappy at having to make new
friends. As she could now drive, however, I did not feel that I
was condemning her to a life of isolation.

With the help of the money I made from selling off the
product side of the recording business, I set about trying to turn
the house into a home-cum-business. The ground floor at one
end of the house I earmarked as an office and healing room.
That needed to be put right first to enable me to start giving
treatment as quickly as possible. Offloading the sales and promotion side of the recording business was a relief as well as a
source of funds. It had been an on-going worry because I had no
clear idea how to manage it properly.

Within a few months of our moving to Sturgeon's Hall,
Christine became pregnant. Jethro was born the day after my
birthday in August 1991. The world he came into was a non-
stop party. The champagne flowed on the day of his birth.
Christine was adamant that she did not want to stay in hospital
and I was allowed to take her home on condition that her GP
and a health visitor kept a close eye on her and Jethro. Eventually
I went back on the road again to give demonstrations and workshops.

A somewhat disturbing incident that occurred around this
time sticks in my mind. One afternoon during my lunch break at
home, the front doorbell rang. When I answered it there was a
slender woman in her mid-thirties standing on the doorstep. She
said she had an appointment with me. I knew precisely who I
was expecting to see that afternoon and this stranger was not
one of them. I said that she must have made a mistake. She told
me that I had sent her a message on a cassette tape of mine she
had bought in Australia. The message said that I was deeply in

love with her and that she should come to England to marry me. I told her, as gently as I could, that I had not sent her any such message, and then closed the door.

Later in the afternoon the woman began banging on the window of my healing room while I was giving treatment. I went out and remonstrated with her, but could not get her to leave. Eventually she wandered off and I thought I had seen the last of her. That evening she came back again and started knocking on the windows of the dining room. I thought, enough is enough and telephoned the police. When they arrived they told me that there was nothing they could do – just being a nuisance did not constitute a criminal offence. However, they did tell her that technically she was trespassing and eventually persuaded her to go.

The following day, back she came. This really irritated me, because she was now disturbing my patients as well as my temper. I did not think it was right that their time with me should be disrupted. I called the police again, and out they came once more. After speaking to her, one of the policemen said, 'I think I can get rid of her, but you're going to have to play ball with her. I'd like you to come out on the village green with me and meet her. I'll act as your witness, but she wants you to tell her, in my presence as a police officer, that you don't love her, you never have loved her, and you never will love her. Then she'll go.'

By this stage I was ready to do anything, so out we went to play this bizarre charade on a deserted village green in the middle of the afternoon.

'I would like you to confirm that you have never met this lady before.'

'I have never seen her in my life. I have never met her.'

'I want you to confirm that you are not in love with her.'

'No, I am not in love with her. I am married.'

'I'd like you to tell me that to the best of your knowledge you are not likely to be in love with her in the future.'

'No, I won't be.'

The woman remained silent thoughout this interchange. At the end of it, she seemed quite happy for the policeman to lead her away. I took her air of resignation as a good sign, but a few hours later she was back at the house. This time the police arrested her. They discovered that she had come from Australia with her fourteen-year-old daughter, and was staying in bed and breakfast accommodation in Bury St Edmunds. She was granted bail, and undeterred by the threat of further arrest immediately returned to Sturgeon's Hall. Christine and I were not made aware of this until much later, when we returned to the house after an evening out.

Christine went straight upstairs to bed, and I let our two dogs out for a run. I came back into the kitchen and there the woman was. I have never experienced such a primeval force as took hold of me the instant I realized that my territory and privacy had been invaded. I was so livid at the fact of her being in the house – and by the idea that she might have been there for several hours – that I acted in a way I regret now but at the time seemed absolutely right. I picked her up and literally threw her out of the back door. The commotion brought Christine downstairs. Unbalanced by suspicion, as soon as she saw the woman she picked up a carving knife and went after her.

Fearful of what might happen, I dialled 999 and reported an intruder. They asked me if the intruder was armed. I said, 'No, but my wife is.' They asked me if I knew the intruder. I said, 'Yes'. An armed response unit arrived at the house within a few minutes of my making that call. I have never seen so many police cars appear from so many directions. I was told that the unit had been on the other side of the village on business totally unconnected with what was happening at my house.

I thought this was the end of the affair until one of the officers informed me that they would not be able to deprive the woman of her liberty without a compelling reason. The idea that I would have to put up with her constantly on my doorstep seemed outrageous. I was very fortunate in being able to call on someone who could help. Tim Webb, a psychiatrist friend, was living only a few hundred yards down the road. He agreed to come up to the house and talk to the police about what could be done. He took the officers through the procedure of getting the woman 'sectioned' under the Mental Health Act. Fortunately for me, they acted on his advice and within a few days she was deported.

✳   ✳   ✳

It is said that we teach what we need to learn. Increasingly, the material I was presenting in my workshops was reflecting my situation with myself. The healing of relationships and the emotional self became the focus of my workshops. I was helping people to find ways of increasing the quality of their lives, maximizing their inner strengths and letting go of all those pent-up negative feelings – anger, guilt, fear.

I knew exactly what I was talking about. The problems I was asking people to confront were my own. I did not have to search for anecdotes and stories of desperate unhappiness to know about the props we use to get us through and deaden the pain. I had my own book of life to read from. This public admission of what is for many people an unpalatable weakness had a polarizing effect.

Many New Agers, appalled that I should have sunk so low, were put off. In their eyes I had taken the spiritual sheen off healing and brought it down to an unacceptably basic level. They were also disappointed in me for not being who they thought I should be – Matthew 'Next to Godliness' Manning. The reality fell too far short and could not be accepted. I was not allowed to be ordinarily human and flawed – to be confused, to be impatient and show anger, to make wrong choices, to have earthly and earthy desires, to admit to having problems.

There were people who could draw strength from my weakness. I started noticing a shift, too, in the balance between the sexes coming to my talks and demonstrations. Previously women had far outnumbered men. Now the 20 per cent increased to 50 per cent as women started bringing husbands, sons and boyfriends. These people were not appalled to hear that I knew all about heavy drinking or about the many difficulties that arise out of personal relationships. Quite the reverse. It made them feel that I was part of the world they inhabited. I was not talking down to them while holding myself up as some paragon. If I had, they would not have listened and wild horses would not have dragged them back to hear me again. I saw virtue in the audience's ability to relate to me. I set healing in a context they could relate to and accept. Many ailments are physical manifestations of unresolved emotional problems, and it was the roots of these that many in my audience wanted to pore over with me. My truthfulness was perceived as a strength, an encouragement to those with a similar problem.

At this time, when Christine and I were not drinking in the local pub, we were holding parties at Sturgeon's Hall, sometimes informal, sometimes lavish when we would have large fireworks displays and blast the neighbourhood with hugely amplified music. The house stank most of the time of alcohol and cigarettes. As there were few furnishings to worry about, this did not matter. Sturgeon's Hall was an ideal shell for people who lived to drink and party, addicted to the image they were cutting. I changed the way I dressed and my look. I grew my hair long, started buying very bright jackets and bought a Bentley that I drove far too fast. I was succeeding in becoming the antithesis of what people expected. It was a hollow triumph. I did not like the person I saw. He was just another image that a boy might want to adopt during his search for himself. Looking back, I wonder who that person was.

The results I was getting with healing, however, remained impressive. Take Inga Olsson, for example. She had attended two healing circles in 1994 shortly after X-rays had identified a malignant tumour attached to her spine as the cause of the excruciating back pain from which she suffered. When she went home after the second circle – filled with energy and positive thoughts, she told me later – the fuses in the house blew the instant she turned on the light. For a couple of days after the circle she felt angry for no particular reason, although still positive. She thought of it as a cleansing, as though something was being released. A bone scan was taken shortly after the circles, and this showed that the tumour had completely disappeared.

I could not argue with such an outcome, and yet it did not seem right that my way of life had no bearing on what I was doing. What was this saying about who I was? I began to wonder if I was a reincarnation of Rasputin, a dissolute possessed of superhuman power or energy. I even bought a book about him to see if there were any similarities.

The discovery that I was not invulnerable came on the night of my thirty-eighth birthday. I had been drinking for hours when suddenly I keeled over and was violently sick. The people in my group thought this was funny, because by this point in my drinking career I had built up a reputation as a very hard man indeed. There were cheers all round that I had at last gone down.

The person who placed me in the crash position to prevent choking probably saved my life, because I could not stop vomiting. I lost consciousness and when I came round it was almost two in the morning. The people still remaining wanted to call an ambulance to take me to hospital. I was in no state to resist but I did not want to have my stomach pumped. The landlord objected too; an ambulance arriving at his door so long after hours might tip off the police.

A doctor I knew was contacted and agreed to come out. After a brief examination, she said I must have my stomach pumped. Again, I resisted. Very reluctantly she agreed not to unilaterally call an ambulance on condition that someone would remain with me and that if I was sick again I would go into hospital. I stayed in the pub until eight in the morning before making my way home. When I stripped off to shower I found bruises, some of them the size of dinner plates, all over my body, signs that my much put upon liver had started to fail.

Those marks of physical mortality frightened me into cutting back. I was in danger of losing control. In my professional life I was moving towards a point where my excesses were feeding my work. This was imposing a terrible strain on me emotionally. Like a worn elastic band stretched to breaking point, something had to give. It almost did in March 1994 at a place called Sundvolden in Norway.

I was at the end of a four-day workshop that had been a highly emotional experience for the people taking part, with outpourings of pent-up grief, regret, sorrow and anger. In the closing moments someone in the audience stood up and thanked me for having been so open. As I listened a tremendous wave of emotion began to well up inside. I was clinging to self-control by my fingernails and would not let go. I turned my back and stood facing the wall for several minutes while I went through every technique I knew to regain my composure.

✳ ✳ ✳

I have often taught that change is the situation most likely to cause us stress because of our perceived inability to adapt to it. Change is cast in the role of demon. The real culprit, though, is that perceived inability; in short, fear. When it comes to relationships, fear is the worst possible 'glue' and yet it can be remarkably enduring. It kept Christine and me clinging to the wreckage for at least five years longer than was good for either of us. Neither of us had the courage to break free. The stagnation of no change was preferable to the unknown. We reached a point, however, where we could no longer ignore the utter futility of our marriage.

I had just completed a week of giving workshops in Sweden and had rung Christine to tell her which flight I was taking and the time she could expect me home. I drove myself from Heathrow Airport and arrived at Sturgeon's Hall at around ten. The car of a farmer friend of Christine's called Edward was in the driveway. I thought nothing of this until I got to the front door and noticed that the house was in darkness. My key would not open the door, which seemed to be locked from the inside. I felt rather annoyed and rang the bell a few times before going round to the back of the house. Why the lights were out and what was going on inside suddenly hit me.

My mind was churning with dark thoughts of what I would do to the pair of them when I walked into the bedroom. I picked up a large wooden mallet and started to go up the stairs. I was almost at the top when a flash of reason brought me up short. I thought, 'If I hit them, I will be the one who pays the price.' I turned around, went back down the stairs and out into the garden, and threw the mallet as far away as my strength would carry it.

I can only conclude that Christine wanted me to find her with Edward. Perhaps it was the only way she could find of crawling out of the pit we had dug for each other. I should have been grateful when she left with Edward. On 25 April 1994, I went to my solicitor to start separation proceedings.

It was eventually agreed that I should rent a cottage for Christine and the children in a nearby village. I had coped with Henrietta and Jethro for the short period after the split when they had been with me, but there was no question in my mind, or Christine's, that they should be looked after by their mother.

The final break with Christine did not bring about a dramatic change in me. I had still a little way to go before the brick wall finally hit me. Two weeks after Christine left I went on a massive twelve-hour drinking binge in the company of an acquaintance who must have had as many demons cluttering up his life as I had cluttering up mine.

Someone took me home. I can remember waking up on the floor. I felt physically wrecked, but my mind would not let me take refuge in that. I needed to come out of this experience with more than a hangover, otherwise I was going to end up killing myself or dying inadvertently. The house was empty. It was just me, enclosed on all sides. I had no audience, no friends, no wife. That is a very alien situation for someone who is rarely totally alone. I played Pink Floyd's album *Division Bell* over and over again. Two lines from one of the tracks kept running through my mind:

I knew the time had arrived
For killing the past and coming back to life.

I wrote the words on dozens of pieces of paper and stuck them to surfaces all over the house – on walls, mirrors and doors. This was my affirmation. It is often said that before you can heal others you have to heal yourself. I think there is quite a lot of truth in this. In my workshops I was teaching the power of affirmative or positive thinking to help overcome fears and lead the self out of retreat. For years I had been urging salvation on others without finding my own. Now it was my turn.

Chapter 6

INTO THE LIGHT

That terrible night forced me to acknowledge that I had to change my way of life, but I had no idea how it would happen. I was like a reckless driver who has caused a near-miss on a motorway – temporarily chastened and all the while fighting the urge to put his foot down hard again. I did not begin to turn my empty vessel round and head it in the right direction until six weeks later, on 7 June, the start of a four-day workshop I was giving in London.

There were fewer people than I expected, about forty. I should not have been surprised. In comparison with other nationalities the British are loath to part with their money for such events. I was standing around watching the people trickle in to the hall and seat themselves in the two rows of chairs arranged in a horseshoe when I was stopped in my tracks. Something clicked in my consciousness, like a flash of recognition. I knew I had been caught by more than the looks of the woman who had come into the room, or what she was wearing – a rather unseasonable combination of long floral dress and black knee-length boots. But, as I would discover, that is Gig.

I have a rule in my workshops that after each break people have to move and sit somewhere else. It is better for the flow of energies if people do not stick together in huddles. I noticed that everybody would shift except for this beautiful woman with blonde hair. It was only later I realized that she had, and it was my perspective that had remained fixed, because I had been reorienting myself to face wherever she was sitting. The only person I noticed during those four days was Gig, and my mind was taken up with figuring out how I could get to talk to her. It was a very frustrating experience. At every break I was surrounded by people and could not get to her before she disappeared from the room.

I did not know it at the time, but Gig was also aware of a connection between us, although she had difficulty identifying its nature. She had been recommended to try healing and had come along full of curiosity, not knowing what to expect. She got more than she bargained for. During the workshop she saw lines of white light darting between us like electricity and heard herself saying that she loved me.

Gig accepted these experiences on the level of spiritual knowledge, and did not associate them with me personally until the end of the four days. Very cleverly, I thought, I asked her if she ever left London. The absence of a 'we' in her reply encouraged me to ask her out. When she came over to say goodbye, I knew I had about fifteen seconds to make a move or run the risk of losing track of her for a long time. I told her that I would be coming back on the 28th for a party at David Frost's London home and would she like to go out for dinner afterwards. When she said 'Yes' and gave me her card, I could hardly conceal my delight.

*   *   *

David Frost has been like a fairy godfather to me, appearing at two critical points in my life to wave a magic wand and make things happen. We did one radio show together shortly after *The Frost Interview* in 1974 and then lost touch until the end of 1993. The call he left on my ansafone was one of the many things passing me by at this time, and it went unanswered. Shortly after Christmas he telephoned again and we arranged to meet in Suffolk.

Over lunch at a local restaurant we discussed a new project that he was in the process of putting together through his company, David Paradine Productions. Would I be interested in co-presenting, alongside himself and Uri Geller, an hour-long television show in which aspects of the paranormal would be investigated live? Carlton Television had bought the package and were proposing to broadcast the show at prime time on a Saturday night in spring 1995.

I did not need time to consider David's offer. I looked upon it as a golden opportunity to further my aspirations for healing and demonstrate its benefits to the widest possible audience. The idea of treating the paranormal as entertainment did not seem an inherent danger. I had always managed to make my own presentations as slick as possible without detracting from the importance of what I was putting across. Television could surely do as well.

Intuitively I did not doubt the seriousness with which David himself viewed the subject. The producer of what would become *Beyond Belief,* Trevor Poots, told me later that the idea for the show was formed after the death of David's mother in 1990, but the seed for it had been planted at the time of *The Frost Interview* we did together. People never forget the things in life that have meaning for them, and David has never forgotten that particular show because it pushed him towards a belief in the paranormal.

Once I was back in David's orbit I was immediately put on his guest list for parties. The party of 28 June was held in the gardens of Carlyle Square. As is my custom, I got there early, ten minutes ahead of the time given on the formal invitation and before the security men had taken up their positions on the gate. I was standing around by myself clutching a drink when a policeman approached me and asked for my name. I suppose it was not surprising that he should have been suspicious of someone who was instantly unrecognizable. David's parties are like visiting Madame Tussaud's and finding that many of the waxwork figures have come to life. His guests come from the worlds of sport, entertainment, business and politics.

After a little while by myself I went round to Gig's flat a few streets away and, wanting to impress her, asked if she would like to have a bit of fun celebrity spotting before we had dinner.

The party was just getting interesting when we arrived. The paparazzi were out in force, risking life, limb and dignity to get into the best shooting positions. The bigger the name the later the arrival, and the louder the whirring of camera shutters.

The party-goers themselves were less worried about focusing only on people they recognized. Gig could have had something to do with this. Paddy Ashdown came up, teeth and eyes glinting, and introduced himself, followed closely by an as keen though plastered Richard Branson, who asked her for a cigarette.

I said, 'I thought you didn't smoke.'

'When I'm drunk, I'll do anything.'

At the end of the party his wife swept past with, 'You can either come with me or stay here.' He tossed the cigarette one way, the glass the other, and exited after her.

The following year, I would glimpse the sober side of Branson. I received a hand-written letter from him, asking if I would give an urgent appointment to the mother of one of his employees who had a brain tumour. Each of his employees is given his home telephone number and knows he can be relied upon to give assistance in a personal emergency. In this case the woman did not take up the appointment offered. When I met Branson again, I thanked him for writing. Not many people in his position are prepared to involve themselves so directly in the well-being of their staff.

Being with Gig seemed totally right from that first night. Prior to her walking into my workshop, I would have vehemently rejected the idea of getting involved in another permanent relationship so soon after splitting with Christine. Intuitively, though, I knew Gig was special and that the feelings she was bringing out in me were too. I wanted to be with her, and invited her to come up to Suffolk the following weekend.

Bad habits, though, are difficult to shake off, even when we have had enough of them. Although I had cut down on the drinking, I was still having more alcohol than was good for me. When Eros came along, he seemed intent on scuppering what was left of my best intentions. The village in which Sturgeon's Hall stands has a limited range of amusements and diversions to offer the visitor. When Gig came up for that first weekend I took her to its social hub, the pub. The Dutch courage flowed and, thoroughly weakened, I told her I had met my match. Then I panicked. It had only been our second date. How unsophisticated to blurt out the truth and risk frightening her off. I tried to 'clarify' the meaning of my remark, explaining that I thought she was a match for me because she could keep up with my partying, that was all.

Two weeks later I was cornered. We were drinking in the pub, again, when in walked a local girl with whom I had been having a casual relationship. I did not wait to make the expected introductions and bundled an indignant Gig into the kitchen out of sight. Having avoided one confrontation, I found another looking at me. Gig was furious and spelled out a few home truths which I was incapable of refuting. I had a straight choice: go on as I was or acknowledge my past, reject it and commit myself to the love that Gig embodied.

A few days later I left on a ten-day tour of Norway. Although Gig said nothing, I sensed that she wanted to go with me and was disappointed when I did not suggest it. I could not bring myself to tell her that I had to go alone to prove to myself that my previous lifestyle no longer held any attraction. I knew from past experience with Christine that it is not difficult to remain faithful when there is no opportunity for anything else. I had to be able to save myself from myself. I did not want Gig as a jailer. I wanted her as a loving equal who could trust me.

My new-found sobriety came as a shock to Walter Kraus, and probably as a relief, too. We spent ten moderately sober, restful nights on the road together. I did not even look at the women around me and my sole concern was whether Gig might find somebody else during my absence.

Over the following weeks I discovered what it is to be one's self. Previously it had seemed as though I had not been allowed to be me. Now that I had been given permission, I could move from being an image to being fully human.

I knew I had been incredibly lucky to find Gig. I had not been able give Christine the love she needed, whereas with Gig it was as easy as breathing. I suppose when we are filled with the indescribable joy love brings, we assume that other people are experiencing something similar in their close relationships. I had been confident that Christine would be as happy with Edward as I was with Gig. Indeed, when I had watched them leave Sturgeon's Hall after turfing them out of my bed, part of me had felt envious of Christine. At bottom, Edward was a thoroughly decent, honourable man who was willing to give her what I could not. Only a few months had passed, however, before I started hearing disturbing stories.

My intake of alcohol dramatically reduced after I met Gig. There were so many more interesting things to do. Christine, though, seemed to be drinking even more, not socially, but in the way that people do when they seem hell-bent on their own destruction and are oblivious of the consequences to themselves or anyone else, including their children. The situation was brought to a head a few days before Gig and I were due to fly to Australia, and mainly on account of Christine's drinking.

I was awarded temporary custody of the children by the courts. I appointed a nanny to look after them at Sturgeon's Hall while I was away. A few months later the children were back living with Christine after she had convinced social workers of her fitness.

* * *

As I changed, I began to notice a corresponding change in the healing, or rather in people's responses to it. This was especially evident in the four-day workshops. The content was the same as before – centring on the unresolved conflicts in our lives and the damage they cause – but people seemed to be affected at a much deeper level.

I remember one workshop in Norway at this time, and one man in particular. He seemed very self-contained until almost the end when he became demented and began retching uncontrollably, as though he was trying to expel something alien from his body. Later I discovered that for over twenty years he had been attempting to come to terms with his sexuality through psychotherapy. During the healing circle he had received a very clear picture of himself as a three-year-old being attacked and then raped by a man.

Years of therapy had failed to uncover this memory and its associated trauma. Its release changed his view of himself and enabled him to discover who he really was. When I saw him again months later, I was struck by how much happier and positive he seemed. He had been transformed by his experience. Even when healing temporarily disturbs, it never works against us.

These workshops, with their emphasis on emotional and spiritual revelation, began to frighten me. They were such highly charged events, and becoming increasingly so. I was beginning to wonder how much more draining they could get. I could not cordon myself off from the emotions being dredged up in others, nor had I wanted to in the beginning. The need to clean out those dark, secret corners of experience had been as much mine as that of the people participating. The time came when the need was no longer there. I had no intimation of it until it happened.

Again, I was in Scandinavia, nearing the end of a five-day workshop. I do not know why, but I had been very close to tears several times during the preceding four days. On the last morning, I began to tell the story of my meeting with Gig. I had not got very far with it when I felt tears streaming down my face. This time I did not turn away to hide them.

The reaction of the ninety people in front of me was extraordinary. There was an empathetic dissolving into tears all around. My emotion, though, was not caused by sadness or distress. It was a manifestation of ineffable happiness, and an acknowledgement that the past was no longer shadowing my life. After five years of teaching the meaning of love, I knew I had found it. The teacher had been taught. He would have to find another lesson.

✳   ✳   ✳

I revised the content of the workshops after this experience, dropping a lot of material and shortening them to one- or two-day events. This had no effect whatsoever on the healing, which will always work at the level of need within each individual. From my own perspective there seemed to be a better balance between the various dimensions, but that was purely because I could now lead and guide unhindered by the personal problems I had been working through. The emotional dimension lost none of its potency, as the following two letters reveal. Anita Ridley wrote:

> Last night you chose to heal me at the workshop in the Festival for Mind, Body and Spirit. I had been so desperate for healing, I had been sending you vibes whilst travelling up on the train to the Festival. Whilst sitting in the audience, I was imagining myself getting up and walking up to you to receive help. However, it happened, you picked me!
>
> I suffered from an eating disorder for many years and had so much hurt and fear trapped inside me that it eventually manifested itself in my lower spine causing osteoarthritis (apparently, unwittingly I was preventing the spinal fluid from flowing in that section of my back when I became distressed) which in turn caused the bone spur growing into my spinal cord. The prolapsed disc occurred as a result of further deterioration in that area. I have also been born with a narrow spinal canal, which made any weakness in that area a real problem.
>
> I had an operation in June 1994 at the Neurosurgical Department in the Brooke Hospital. I had been left with scarring both internally and externally and had considerable nerve pain in my legs. I also had my lower spine fused.
>
> During the healing you gave me, the hurt came to the surface and freed itself . . . I felt you drawing the hurt out into your hand like white streams of light flowing out of

my legs through the centre of my lower back. You send out so much comfort and love when you are healing, you become magnetic. I have never experienced so much intense feeling from a human being. I believe you have powers far beyond 'human' capabilities. I know your healing process continued with me throughout last night. I felt the process so strongly it kept me awake for hours!

You said that you saw the colours green and yellow whilst working with me. My bedroom is green and yellow and is the one place where I feel completely safe and 'me'. Whether or not you picked this up, I don't know.

I feel wonderful. My back feels free and flexible. I feel that my legs have undergone and are still undergoing a transformation, freeing themselves and continuing to heal. They are pain-free and my feet are still tingling. I had been restricted, depressed and uncomfortable for so long that it feels sensational being able to touch my toes again. Indeed, once last night, I have touched my toes at least ten times because it feels so good. Quite how I am able to do that with a fused, arthritic back, I don't know!'

The second letter read as follows:

I recently attended one of your healing circles in Exeter. I found the experience deeply moving and thought that you might like to hear about it. I came to see you for two reasons. The first is because I have been trying for a child for over seven years. The second was because I have also had ME for the last three of those years, and although better than I was, I felt very trapped in a cycle of stress and illness.

Sitting in the circle I had no idea what to expect. I am quite alternative and 'green' but not a very 'esoteric' person, which made what happened all the more surprising to me. I tried to just let go into the beautiful music and this is where I went . . .

First, I was sitting on my sofa at home. I became smaller and smaller until I turned into a white bird – a gull maybe. I flew out of the window and into the sky. At this point I thought maybe I would have a feeling of freedom and lightness – maybe this is what I needed – but no. I flew directly off up the A38 towards the east. I felt in control but not of where I was going. I just followed. It soon became very clear I was flying to London, over all the familiar landmarks that I knew so well.

As I reached London, the journey became more and more detailed. Across the streets of west London, past Euston, King's Cross, up to Islington and on to Hackney – the route I have always taken. And then I was there, circling above my parent's house, the house I grew up in. I could see myself aged seven or eight. I was standing in the cold, bleak hall by myself. I knew that I had to fly down and contact this child but was prevented from doing so by a wall of pain so vast that I thought it would break my heart. I don't think I have ever cried so deeply (and I have cried a lot before). My heart just hurt so much. Someone then came and touched me (one of the healers who was helping you). I immediately felt a wave of calmness wash over me and in this I was able to fly down and meet and then become this child.

(At this point it might be helpful to know that, as a child, I received almost no physical or emotional love from either parent.) Standing in the hall (as a child) I felt very unhappy. Desolate and not knowing what to do, the words 'Why don't you love me?' went round and round my head. (As an adult, I have known for a long time about this lack of love and have done lots of work about getting angry with my parents but I have never remembered how I actually felt as a child – just what happened.)

I wandered around the cold house wondering what I should do. Then it seemed that I was the bird again. And I could see that it really wasn't the child's fault that its parents didn't love it. That the child was a beautiful and lovely child who deserved to be loved. That it hurt and it was bad luck that the parents couldn't love it but that it WASN'T the child's fault – how could it be? And then I took the child and together, as two birds, we flew back over the dirty streets of London, on and on and on until we reached Devon.

As we reached the sofa, we turned back into people – it felt very strange – like a big me and a little me. (At this point you put your hands on my shoulders.) I cuddled the little me and gradually she sort of disappeared into the big me. And suddenly as I write this, I realise for the first time in my life that this is probably what people mean when they talk about 'Loving yourself' – I have never really got it before.

Afterwards I felt very vulnerable, but in a really nice way. I still feel very tired and want a baby but I feel as if I have been given some tools to work with now. I gave you a kiss and said thank you but it wasn't enough. So thank you again.

* * *

The production meetings for Paradine's paranormal spectacular got underway in the winter of 1994. I had briefly met Uri Geller in 1988 when he had asked me to appear on a Sunday night show he was giving at London's Prince of Wales Theatre, sponsored by Capital Radio. I was in effect his warm-up man, charged with the task of spending half an hour amusing the audience with stories about healing. He came across as a very strange man, painfully thin, nervy and unable to focus on one activity or idea for longer than a few seconds.

Uri seemed less hyper and disturbed when I met him again, but not to any comforting degree. For every meeting Uri and his manager, Shipi (who is also his brother-in-law), would arrive at David's office in a flurry of noise, conspicuously late, complaining

about the traffic. It is unfortunate for the people who have to wait
for him that Uri's psychic ability does not enable him to foresee the
problems that invariably prevent him arriving anywhere on time.
He would then race over to the nearest window and fling it open
to minimize his exposure to David's large Havana cigars and my
more modestly sized cigarettes. All the *Beyond Belief* shows were
made for broadcast in the spring, so our production meetings took
place in the depths of winter.

Uri's adherence to a purity of lifestyle that would give me
nightmares probably went some way towards insulating him from
the effects of the icy blasts gusting around the room. He was
helped too by his inability to remain still for longer than a couple
of seconds at a time. He would be jogging on the spot, jumping
up and down or off the furniture, or pacing around the room.

I find it very difficult to think straight when someone is per-
petually moving around me and virtually impossible when they
are simultaneously carrying on a conversation with someone else
about a totally unconnected topic. David would always make a
point of not taking calls for the duration of the meeting. Not so
Shipi, who would be sitting there wired for sound, wearing an
earpiece plugged into his mobile phone. Our three-way conversation about the show would take place against the backdrop of
Shipi constantly making or receiving calls, and asking Uri for
instructions.

The biggest problem we hit during the planning stages was
finding other people with paranormal abilities who would be
prepared to demonstrate them without the safety net of prefilm-
ing. The show had to be totally live to be credible. This approach
was also intended to give the proceedings 'edge' – too much it
seemed for the 'names' we approached in Britain, every one of
whom turned us down. We were forced to look much farther
afield – to Russia for Uri's 'find', mind-reader Boris Tulchinsky,
and the United States for mine, fire-walker Christina Thomas.
The easy bit was deciding what Uri and I should do.

I agreed to perform a mind/body exercise and healing
demonstration. For the healing demonstration I asked the

production team at Paradine to find somebody with restricted movement and a high level of pain. I felt sure that what works for a live audience in a hall would work for a live audience in a television studio. I knew that I was fairly good at knocking out pain quickly, and the performer in me knows that televisually it is very effective to show the effect healing can have on someone with restricted movement: before healing they cannot lift their arm above shoulder height and after it the arm can be raised above head height. After making enquiries among various doctors, the researchers faxed me a list of fourteen people to choose from.

I ran my eyes down the list and waited for one of the names to push itself forward. When this happened, I knew I had found the person I should use. The woman was in her mid-thirties and had spinal injuries from a serious car crash two years previously. More distressing than the considerable pain caused by her injuries was her inability to lift her small child. She could not bend, turn her head or raise her arms. Intuitively, I knew the healing would work with her. I asked one of the researchers to call the woman and check that she would be able to give a good account of herself on television. A few hours later the researcher called me back and said the woman was ideal: she had a clear speaking voice, and was eloquent and positive.

On the day before the broadcast the woman telephoned Paradine and told them she would have to pull out. An insurance claim against the driver of the other car involved in the accident that had resulted in her injuries was pending and her solicitor had advised her of the possible adverse consequences of her appearing on the show. The payment she was expecting would be greatly reduced if she was seen to be pain-free and mobile after the healing demonstration.

It was beyond my comprehension that a person who was undoubtedly experiencing considerable physical and emotional pain should be prepared to forfeit an opportunity to rid herself of them for the sake of money. But there was not time to philosophise. Blind panic took over. We had to find a suitable placement. I asked the researcher to invite the thirteen other people on the list to the studio of Central Television in Nottingham so I could make another choice.

The following day at around lunchtime I walked into the room where they were all gathered and introduced myself. Within a few minutes I knew which of them to choose – a man in his fifties called Keith. I warmed to him immediately. As a child Keith had suffered from Perthes' disease, which affects the hip and is due to fragmentation of the spongy extremity of the tip of the thigh bone. Medical textbooks state that spontaneous recovery from this disorder occurs after a couple of years, but in Keith's case it had left him with arthritis of the lower spine and a restriction between his shoulder blades which he described as 'very painful'.

I was sure I would be able to do something for Keith. In order to make the demonstration more interesting, and also in an attempt to help a few more people for taking the trouble to travel to Nottingham, I selected three others – two women and a man – with problems of restricted movement to join Keith in the demonstration. Thus far with the show the pressure had all been off-camera. On-camera everything went according to schedule.

As presenters Uri and I are as dissimilar as two people can be. My jackets are much louder than my personality, while Uri's dress sense seems to have given up trying to keep pace with his hyper-activity. Understandably the producers of the show wanted to grab the audience's attention at the outset with something which fitted the description of the programme's title, *Beyond Belief.* Uri had tasked himself with involving the audience directly in experiments with psychokinesis and telepathy. He whirred around the studio organizing these mass experiments. The first involved broken watches, which a large number of the 300-strong audience had brought with them to the studio, spoons and keys.

Everyone, including people watching the programme at home, was asked to concentrate on getting the broken watches to start working again and keys and spoons to bend. Watching Uri work is an experience – perhaps the phrase watching him 'be' is more appropriate. I have never come across anyone who can generate that much energy outside his own body. It can be disturbing. When everybody was asked to shout 'Work', loudly and meaningfully on a count of three, no one in the studio shouted more loudly or meaningfully than Uri. In a matter of seconds some of the broken watches started ticking and people were holding them out for examination.

My mind/body exercise made a similar point to Uri's about how energy can be used. In his demonstration energy was being directed outwards at objects. In my mind/body exercise I wanted to show how different kinds of thought can affect the body and, most importantly, our ability to resist. The exercise was one I had used many times in public demonstrations, as a 'step one' of healing. The impressively bronzed and muscled Panther, from the television show *Gladiators*, was there to assist me.

After ascertaining that the right side of her body was stronger than the left, I asked her to think for about fifteen seconds of something that made her feel very happy, inspired and positive. When she felt she had absorbed this idea, she was to put out her left arm and when I said the word 'Resist', she was to use every ounce of her strength to prevent me pushing her arm down. I was virtually jumping on her arm, but could not bring it down to the side of her body.

We repeated the exercise on her right side, only this time I asked her to change her frame of mind and think of something that made her feel angry, hostile, jealous and negative. Being on her stronger side, her right arm looked even more formidable than her left, and yet it collapsed as soon as I exerted pressure on it. Panther could find no explanation for what happened to her. It is very simple: anyone can be humbled by negative thoughts – even someone who has a body that is in peak physical condition – or made stronger by positive ones.

Healing makes bad television, as riveting as watching paint dry unless you happen to be one of the people taking part. It is also a very personal activity, which people have to give themselves up to. After each of the participants had been introduced ne audience and had their ailments described, I took them to a room near the studio where they would be more likely to relax and create an atmosphere conducive to healing. As Keith was the one to whom I felt most attuned and he had two very obvious restrictions, I chose to work on him directly. I arranged all four of the participants in a circle, linking hands, and began to work.

I had ten minutes to make a difference, or not, half the time I usually allow for a demonstration. At the end of it we returned to the main studio. I studiously avoided asking any of them how they felt until we were back in front of the cameras. However, I had an idea as to which of them had benefited – although how is always another matter – and was particularly curious to discover how effective the healing had been for Keith. Before the healing session all four had demonstrated their immobility to the audience and been checked over by a physiotherapist, who had verified their stated incapacity.

I did not hold out much hope for the healing helping the disability of one of the women, whose neck bones had been fused by surgery. Her immobility was as fixed as before, although she did report feeling more relaxed and being free of the headache she had had before the session. The other woman also said she felt more relaxed. The most striking result was with the two men. Peter was suffering from an arthritic shoulder, which prevented him making lateral or vertical movements with his arm. He said he had felt the energy passing around the circle and could now demonstrate considerably more mobility than previously.

But the most striking improvement was seen in Keith. He described the healing as an 'incredible experience' and said he had felt the pain leaving his body. He could now raise his arms above his head, and his ability to bend over at the waist was much improved because the pain in his lower spine had lessened.

At the party after the show, Keith expressed his gratitude for having been chosen for the healing. He told me a story:

> When I first heard that you were looking for somebody as
> a demonstration subject on the show, I started to imagine
> that it was going to be me. I imagined what it would be
> like to be under your hands. I imagined myself being pain-
> free. I could feel the heat. Then I discovered I was on the
> shortlist. But then I did not hear any more. At this point
> I started redoubling my efforts. I have been carrying
> around a photograph for the last week. On the hour, every
> hour, I have been getting this photograph out and looking
> at it and imagining myself being the person on that tele-
> vision show, being healed. I've got the photograph with
> me.

He pulled it out of his pocket and showed me a photograph of
myself.

Keith's story about how he came to receive healing reminded
me of a similar incident ten years previously. On that occasion I
had asked for a volunteer during a demonstration at the Healing
Arts Exhibition in London. That evening there were only two
people – a man and a woman – I could work with, both of
whom had locked necks. I asked if there was a physiotherapist
in the audience who would check the disability of both people
and make the choice for me. (In those days I would regularly
make this request, purely to underline to the sceptical or suspicious that the demonstration was genuine and the subjects were
not paid accomplices.) The woman who stepped forward
examined the two and then opted for me to work with the man.
This put me in a quandary because intuitively I knew I should
work with the woman and yet I could not be seen to refuse the
choice made for me.

The woman and the physiotherapist returned to their seats
in the audience and I set to work on the man. After about fifteen
minutes, I thought I was going to ignite with heat. Something
was happening, I felt sure. I continued for a few more minutes
and then asked him if there was any improvement in his neck.
He tried moving it, but it was still locked as solidly as it had been

...he start of the session. I was completely baffled, because I knew some profound change had occurred. I was pondering this when my attention was drawn to a commotion in the audience. The woman to whom I had wanted to give the healing was standing up. She had removed the surgical collar which she had been wearing, and was shouting, 'Look' as she turned her neck in all directions, without restriction or pain.

This experience – and Keith's – suggests that healing will find its intended recipient, even when obstacles are put in its way, albeit inadvertently or unwittingly. In Keith's case I had initially chosen someone else, but she had taken herself out of the equation at the last minute, leaving the way clear for him. The same explanation can be applied to the incident at the Healing Arts Exhibition. The healing was intended for that woman and even though my hands were on the man, the energy found its way to her.

A couple of weeks after finishing *Beyond Belief* I went to Sweden to work, accompanied by Walter and Gig. We spent some of this ten-day trip in the small town of Bollnas within the Arctic Circle. The place was so small we had to be flown in by a light aircraft. Our hotel provided all the usual comforts except one – food at critical times of the day. It would give us breakfast but after that we were thrown on our own resources.

This would not have mattered if we were in a country where restaurants and other eating places are in abundance, but in Sweden outside the major centres they are very thin on the ground. It is little wonder that Swedish cuisine is not known around the world when it is barely detectable in its own country. For the hungry traveller in Sweden there are no immigrant cuisines to make up the shortfall either. I would start work at ten in the morning with healing circles which went on all day. In the evening I would give a workshop that would start at six o'clock and finish around ten. Then we would begin the trudge through the freezing cold, dark, damp streets looking for something edible. I have never been so glad to leave a place.

A few days after Gig and I arrived home, I had a vivid dream. In it I was watching the Grand National steeplechase and listening to the commentary. As the horses passed the winning post, I could hear the commentator shouting excitedly, 'And the winner is Mr Cinnamon.' Then the dream switched from the race to that town in the north of Sweden. It is cold, dark and I am very hungry. I am with Walter and together we are wandering the streets looking for a restaurant. Everywhere is in darkness. One restaurant we pass is boarded up. Then ahead of us I see a warm, golden glow of light shining onto the pavement from an open doorway.

We reach the doorway and discover it is the entrance to a night-club and there are steps leading down to it. I say 'Great. There must be food in here.' Then I realize that we are unlikely to get in because neither of us is a member. Walter, whose nickname is 'No Problem', produces a card from his pocket and says, 'No problem. I've got membership.' As we go down the steps, Walter turns to me and, with a look that I used to know very well, says, 'Now you can be a real sinner man.'

At this point I became aware of the fact that I was dreaming and made the connection between his turn of phrase and the name of the horse. The dream then ended.

I knew the National was due to be run in a couple of days' time, and my first thought on waking the next morning was to check the list of runners. When I could find neither a Mr Cinnamon nor a Sinner Man, I decided that perhaps I had been too quick to read significance into the dream. Yet it had been so clear, so lucid, unusually so. I went through into my office where my secretary was just coming in with the post. It was unusually heavy, about 400 letters, because a few days earlier an article about me had appeared in the *Daily Mail*. The Post Office had helpfully bundled the letters into batches of fifty, fastened with elastic bands.

My secretary put the bundles on the table and because my first patient was either late or did not turn up, I decided to open some of the letters. I do not often get this opportunity and always find it interesting when I do. I picked up one of the bundles and pulled out an envelope at random. The letter I had chosen was from someone who said he had known about my work for a long time but had not known how to get in touch with me. Then he had seen the article in the *Daily Mail*, which had included my address. He was requesting information about workshops and how he should go about getting one-to-one healing with me. To my amazement the letter was signed by a Mr Cinnamon of London.

There are several possible explanations. The 'rational' explanation is that old standby 'coincidence' – there is no connection between my dreaming about Mr Cinnamon/sinner man and subsequently receiving a letter from him. Alternatively, was I being clairvoyant in the dream, 'knowing' I was going to open a letter signed by Mr Cinnamon that influenced the dream? I doubt it. My preferred explanation draws on Keith's experience. Had Mr Cinnamon been thinking about me for a few weeks, turning over in his mind what he would like to say to me in his letter? If he had done this and put great creative energy into writing the letter, that energy might somehow have been released into the ether for me to pick up. I spend so much of my time in a meditative state, and 'open' to this kind of communication, it is quite conceivable Mr Cinnamon could have 'tuned in' to me.

In order to accept this explanation, one has to view time in a different way from the norm. Time is for me like trying to contemplate what is beyond the edge of the universe. There are many possibilities that lie beyond the man-made constructs we know as time. Essentially, there is no such thing as time, and it is possible to experience shifts in it when we enter an altered state of consciousness, for instance when dreaming or during meditation – you can go forwards in time and get a premonition or you can go back in time and get a sense of déjà vu.

Imagine time as a compact disc with all actions and thoughts – past, present and future – embedded in its surface as hundreds of thousands of tiny signals. Which of these we pick up and hear through the speakers will depend entirely on the position of the laser on the surface of the disc. We perceive reality to be whatever is happening to us at an instant in time. For most people time moves in only one direction, forwards, like the compact disc which has been programmed to play from track one through to the end. If we are able to move our consciousness back and forth – like that laser – then we can experience different 'tracks' in different time frames.

I first started thinking about time slips when Robert Webbe became known to me. A simple explanation for his 'appearance' would be that he is a dead soul who has not moved on to where he should be. He is, in effect, stuck here, perhaps bound by an over-fondness for material things. A more complex explanation, which I favour, is that time is multi-dimensional and that what Robert Webbe thinks is 4 October 1740 is simultaneously 6 August 1998 or 23 February 2036, or whatever. Perhaps we are living many different lives simultaneously in different time realities. We may be multi-dimensional beings and it may be that our soul or spirit inhabits different bodies at different times in different places.

A person does not have to die to be seen as a ghost. There are well-documented instances of the living being seen in places where it was a physical impossibility for them to be. Mickey Hart, the Grateful Dead's drummer, told me one such story. Behind his ranch house in California there is quite a steep hill of pasture land on which he used to graze horses. The medicine man Rolling Thunder would often come over to the ranch to select some of the herbs growing on that hill for use in his preparations.

One morning Mickey was looking out of his kitchen window when he saw Rolling Thunder on his hands and knees pulling out a plant on the hill. When he looked again a few minutes later, Rolling Thunder was nowhere to be seen. Mickey expected that his friend would shortly appear at the kitchen door and come in for a chat and a coffee, but he did not set eyes on him again that day. He discovered later that Rolling Thunder was 2,000 miles away, treating somebody who, the medicine man knew, needed the plant Mickey had watched him pull from the ground. Rolling Thunder could not physically obtain the plant he needed and so he reached it by means of an intense thought.

The imprint left by thoughts and actions may be negative as well as positive. Dutch healer and clairvoyant Gerard Croiset believed that such energy could be responsible for causing some stretches of road to become accident black spots. His theory was that an enormous burst of energy released in the first crash would subsequently affect other drivers and cause them to have an accident too. Driving is a right-hemispheric activity and some drivers – perhaps those who can slip easily into a meditative state – unwittingly tune into the same energy released traumatically on that spot previously and repeat the mistake made by that first driver. Croiset claimed he could 'heal' these black spots by dispersing the energy at the sites. In several cases the police reported that the accidents stopped after he had worked at a black spot.

*   *   *

Carlton Television received over two and a half million calls from viewers during the transmission of *Beyond Belief* in 1995, and the telephone system in Scotland collapsed through sheer overload. Many of the calls were about spoons and keys bending, broken watches ticking and similar effects achieved by the psychokinetic energy whipped up by Uri. The station also received calls from people who said they had received the benefit of the healing in their own homes while watching the programme.

For me personally the show was a success. As usual, it was Uri who attracted most of the brickbats, with a few specially poisoned darts aimed at David for being so easily impressed.

Some reviewers reserved their comments for what I was wearing rather than attempt to explain the healing. The *Daily Express* thought my jacket should have carried a government health warning.

One of the letters I received in my postbag in the week after the show was from a Mr W.G. Owen. He had been impressed by what he had seen me doing with Peter and wanted to know if I could do the same for his wife, Margaret, who had a number of associated health problems – lumbar scoliosis, degenerative disease of the lower lumbar discs, osteoporosis and artificial hips – which severely restricted her mobility and caused her considerable pain, especially in her spine.

When Mrs Owen first came to see me she told me that she had been sleeping in an armchair for years because the pain and discomfort of sleeping in bed was too great. I felt that if any improvement was to be achieved, it would be slow and probably limited to reducing the high level of pain she was experiencing. I treated her one to one in my practice. A year later her orthopaedic surgeon was reportedly 'very pleased with her condition'. A year on from that, she was at last able to lie down and sleep in her own bed. And in August 1998, he wrote: 'As a scientist, I have to admit I am amazed by how you have become and though there are considerable difficulties, it does look as though an intervention outside of orthodox medicine has come to your aid.'

The viewing figures achieved by the first *Beyond Belief* – over twelve million – encouraged Carlton to plan a similar show for the following year and extend its duration to ninety minutes. An executive at Carlton had decreed that the programme should be 'interactive', and all the features had to be designed with this in mind.

In their eagerness to attract viewers, and through them advertising revenue, Carlton imposed interactivity of a kind that people could expect from a game show, with phone-ins and video links to distant sites. It was circus time – thrills and possibly spills without so much as a thought given to what any of it might mean. There was to be no attempt to ask pertinent questions or get people to think about what was happening in front of them. David's original concept seemed to have been lost and the show suffered as a consequence, not least because of the negativity this shift downmarket engendered.

Uri relished Carlton's insistence on him 'hosting' the many quiz games they were demanding, but even he could not make work what would not. One elaborate telepathy experiment fell flat because of malfunctioning equipment; this had been set up to measure the attempt of a cyclist to break his own world speed record, aided by the combined mind power of Uri, the studio audience and viewers at home. The two guests – Oren, a phenomenal young Israeli who could 'see' telepathically through his father's eyes, and a Polish refugee living in Germany, Miroslav Magala, who had a talent for attaching metal objects to his body – did not repeat the brilliant performances they had given during their auditions.

I felt marginalized, not least because what I was doing was viewed as rather second-rate in the entertainment stakes, an interactive dud. Reluctantly, I agreed to pitch one of my tents with the rest of them, and gave one healing demonstration in the studio while close by the aptly named 'Magnetic Pole' was noisily attracting saucepans and other kitchenware to his body.

I remember being aware of the mayhem around me and not being confident that Barbara, the woman I was working on, would benefit from the healing. She had lost her sense of smell as a result of a sinus infection forty years earlier. The degree of loss was considerable, as she demonstrated immediately before the healing began. Her expression had not so much as flickered when several bottles containing the most penetrating odours imaginable were passed under her nose.

One of these bottles, containing smelling salts, nearly took David's head off when he sniffed at it inquisitively. After twelve minutes of healing, it nearly took Barbara's off too, and she came close to falling off her chair as she recoiled from the smell. David described it as 'an absolutely thrilling moment' and was even more thrilled when at the party after the show Barbara expressed her joy at being able to taste chicken again after so many years.

I had a 'circle' of nine people, including Keith from the first *Beyond Belief*, for my second healing demonstration. Both Keith and Peter, the two who had derived most from the healing given on the first show, had been invited back to report on their progress during the intervening twelve months. Peter said that the

improvement in his condition had continued since the healing
and he was now back to normal. To show how well he now
felt, he lifted both arms above his head and vigorously clapped
his hands together.

Keith had experienced six weeks of freedom from the severe
pain in his lower back, which had been such a burdensome
feature of his problem. However, the pain had gradually crept
back and he was now as afflicted as he had been before the first
show. Given the severity of his condition, this did not surprise
me. Such cases usually require regular healing over many
months. I was hopeful, however, that he would be able to gain
some, albeit probably temporary, relief again by participating in
the healing circle.

I had insisted upon the healing circle being held in private
away from the main studio and so off we went to start the
session. I had been working about three minutes when one of
the studio runners came in and told me we were needed on the
set again. I knew exactly what my schedule was and by my reck-
oning I had another eighteen minutes with the group. My
protestations were brushed aside by the runner, who insisted
that we should all leave immediately and go with her.

When we reached the main studio she realized she had made
a mistake, so we stood in the wings wasting the eighteen minutes
that should have been spent productively in the healing circle. I
tried not to show my anger and frustration when the time came
for us to step forward and report on what had happened.

Needless to say, with so little time having been spent on the
healing, nothing much had happened. At least Keith was able to
say that the pain in his back had begun to drain away and how
much better he felt for that. But all round it was a disappointment, and my feelings reflected wider misgivings about the show
as a whole. I had to say something that might scrape off some of
the cheap gloss Carlton had been eagerly smearing all over it. As
the credits were about to roll, I said: 'You at home might see this
as entertainment, but please also be aware that there are
powerful and positive uses to which energy can be put.'

I was still fuming as I came off the set. It was fitting that the first person I should meet was the executive whose insistence on relentless 'interactivity' had, to my mind, undermined the programme's credibility. I abused him with a tirade that expressed precisely, if inelegantly, my view of him and the company he represented.

*   *   *

Beyond Belief generated a whole new audience for me virtually overnight. The number of people coming to my public events became so large that the local organizations and groups who had previously handled them could no longer do so efficiently. Graham Wilson was the obvious person to put the operation onto a professional footing, and he arranged the annual British tours I undertook from 1995 onwards. These tours were a mixture of a lecture with a healing demonstration or day-long workshops to teach people to develop their own healing abilities.

In addition, I continued my regular 'hops' to Scandinavia, where the interest in healing was as firm as ever. Many people become 'regulars' and will make a point of attending my workshops. Some, like Tatjana Kaufmann, from Naerum in Denmark, retain some element of the experience, in her case by integrating an exercise into her daily routine. A few months after attending one of my seminars, in the Norwegian town of Gausdal, a congenital cyst was discovered attached to her heart valve. Fortunately this cyst was benign, but it could not be removed and it was growing. Tatjana promised herself that if she could not get rid of it, she would contact me.

We had our first healing session together in May 1996. In December of that year the hospital confirmed the cyst had not formed any new tissue and that it had stopped posing a threat to vital organs. By May 1997 the cyst was much reduced and in January 1998 she wrote to say that the hospital felt it was no longer necessary to monitor her. For the moment she is opting to come for healing once a year to maintain the apparently favourable change in her condition.

Nineteen-year-old Laplander Ann Helene Strandgård decided to put off going to college for a year to enable her to come to England for regular healing. In May 1995 she had derived benefit from a series of healing circles and a seminar I had given in the Swedish town of Bollnas and was determined to receive one-to-one healing from me. Ann Helene had cerebral palsy, which in her case was principally characterized by paralysis of the leg muscles and bad balance. Her rather strange walking style imposed great strain on her back, hips and knees and she also experienced great difficulty in concentrating.

As a small child Anne Helene had undergone two operations aimed at lengthening the tendons in her heels to compensate for the paralysis in her calf muscles. These operations enabled her to walk, after a fashion, but as she grew older the abnormal tension in her legs grew more intense and caused her considerable pain. Her first recollection of this pain was as a five-year-old, although her parents told her that she had probably had it since birth as she used to cry too much and sleep too little. This pain had grown worse in the past four years, a symptom which her doctors disregarded because she was the only patient with the condition who complained of it. She declined muscle-relaxants because of their side-effects, which would have necessitated her giving up driving. She was told that if she continued walking as much as she did in her daily life, she would have to accept that within five to ten years she would be wheelchair bound.

Anne Helene visited me for the first time in November 1996 and had three sessions. After each one she had a terrible headache for an hour or two, and after the final session she felt dizzy and sick. In January 1997 she wrote to tell me that the pain had disappeared shortly after the third session:

> This Christmas and New Year have been the happiest in the last seven years of my life. . . . My day-to-day life is easier now. My balance is better. I can move my legs and

my feet, especially the left one, more and I've better control over them now. Before I wrote slowly, but now I am able to write as fast as a healthy person. It's easier to put on and take off my clothes now. I can also walk longer now than before.

The only pain I have left is in the hips and the knees, but I don't have it as often as before the healing and the pain is reduced. I don't have any pain in my back anymore.

The pain in her hips reduced after a second visit, in April 1997, when she experienced 'a strange, burning pain' which moved around in her body. In September 1997 she wrote to me: 'My life has changed since I saw you in November last year. I don't think a human being who has never had chronic pain understands what it means and how relieved I am that it is much less now.'

Ann Helene is now training to help disabled children. The experience of healing has not only enabled her to cope with a major handicap but has resulted in a change of attitude towards herself and life in general.

*   *   *

Television companies, like publishers, always seem to be on the lookout for a bandwagon to jump on to. The first *Beyond Belief* seemed to encourage programme makers from other channels to exploit the paranormal. While the second *Beyond Belief* was in production I was asked by the BBC to do a half-hour video diary of my work. I do not know if the idea for this was prompted by cost-cutting zeal or a genuine belief that a 'home movie' is more revealing of a person than a properly structured film.

It seemed simple enough. I was to take this cine-camera around everywhere and let it record my daily life. The reality left me feeling paralysed and at a loss and every time I tried to use

it, I could not. After my experience of broadcasting and live audiences, I could by no stretch of the imagination be described as
media shy and there are times when I positively relish being in
front of an audience. However, I was far too inhibited for this
exercise. In the end the BBC were forced to get one of their staff
to follow me around and 'shoot' what she thought was interesting. The result, *Order from Chaos*, was one of the few films about
me that I like.

On one occasion during the editing of this film the BBC very
kindly sent a car with a driver to pick me up and take me to
their offices in White City. The driver obviously knew who I was
and we started chatting about *Beyond Belief*. Towards the end of
the journey, he said: 'I'm not going to charge the BBC for this
trip. I have had the most terrible arthritis in my shoulder for the
last three years. I have taken all sorts of things for it. The doctor's
done all sorts of things. None of them has worked. I couldn't lift
my arm. The pain was there constantly. Look at it now.' He
showed me what he meant by moving his arm in all directions.

Two months after *Beyond Belief 2* went out 'live', *Order from
Chaos* was broadcast as part of the BBC series 'Secrets of the
Paranormal'. The film attracted more than its fair share of criticism
for the fact that I had been given complete editorial control. The
argument seemed bogus. All of the previous participants in the
series had exercised complete editorial control by deciding upon
which aspects of their lives they were willing to point that mini-
camera at. I had no more control because the BBC agreed to
second somebody from the Video Diaries unit to help me. Quite
the reverse.

The presence of an outside eye, as it were, made the film
more of a collaboration than a portrait devised solely by me. It
was my intention to correct some of the misconceptions that
people attach to healing. Certainly, I was at pains not to present
myself as some miracle worker. The worst attack was launched
by Professor Lewis Wolpert, Chairman of Copus (the Committee
on the Public Understanding of Science), in a piece he wrote for
the Hypotheses column of the *Independent on Sunday*.

> Matthew Manning, a self-proclaimed healer, repeatedly
> claimed his special powers had been investigated and con-
> firmed by scientists. He even said he could influence cancer
> cells and make medical diagnoses with minimal effort. If
> this were true it would rank as a wonderful new scientific
> discovery: radioactivity, X-rays and radio waves would look
> very pale by comparison. . . . Manning has, of course, no
> such powers. If he had, the so-called scientists who inves-
> tigated him would be rushing into print in the leading
> scientific journals, *Nature* and *Science*, with their findings.

A Dr Denis MacEoin penned a neat riposte to Wolpert's diatribe, which was printed in a subsequent edition of the paper. What depressed me about Wolpert's piece was its shoddiness. It seemed to miss the point entirely, deliberately I suspect, for how many men of Wolpert's undoubted intellect can bear to admit they are at a loss to explain something? They have an argument that the facts have to be made to fit, and will even resort to distorting the truth to ensure it prevails.

Wolpert stated that I claimed to be able to make medical diagnoses. I have never used this ability in my professional work as a healer and indeed will not accept patients for one-to-one healing if their condition has not been identified by a qualified medical practitioner. I had to be a liar and a fraud because he refused to accept the existence of evidence to verify my 'claims'. It would not have taken much research to find the relevant documentation. So much for the frequent boast that the arguments against the existence of paranormal activity are based on an objective, rational pursuit of truth. The worst aspect of his attack, though, was the little importance it attached to the word of people helped by healing.

Roger Adams, one of my patients interviewed for the programme, said:

> I don't feel like a man that's dying. I live the same sort of
> life that I lived six months ago. Although I am supposed

> to have a tumour in my stomach that is the size of a fist,
> I have no problems eating or drinking. I'm a bit short of
> breath, I guess, but that is mainly due to the fact that I
> weigh close on 300 pounds.

Roger was suffering from metastatic cancer in the stomach and liver and, having declined chemotherapy five months earlier, had been given a maximum life expectancy of three months by his consultant oncologist at the Royal Marsden Hospital. Two months after the consultant's prognosis, Roger's liver was deteriorating badly and taking a long time to process fluids. Roger noticed this because, cancer or no, he was determined to enjoy life, and would not give up drinking large quantities of beer.

Roger visited me for the first time about a month later, in January, and after a couple of days he became aware of an improvement in the functioning of his liver. Alcohol that had been taking between twenty-four and forty-eight hours to get though his system was now passing through normally. Roger detailed this in a letter to Wolpert. He also described his experience of the effect of healing on pain:

> During February my wife and I were invited to a Healing
> Circle at the BBC's offices in Wood Lane. About forty
> people turned up. I cannot be certain, but I assume that
> the group comprised twenty patients and their compan-
> ions. My wife had suffered from a chronic pain in her
> spine: a condition which sometimes accompanies the
> menopause, described as osteoporosis.
>
> I had woken up that morning with the very first serious
> intimation of the pain that liver cancer can cause. The
> journey facing us comprised a bus trip, three changes of
> Tube train, followed by a long walk, and I've got to tell
> you, we were mightily reluctant to go. Nevertheless, we
> didn't want to let anyone down, and so we forced our-
> selves to set out.
>
> After we arrived, we were formed into a circle and

cautioned against breaking it. By this time I was sweaty and nauseous and in a great deal of pain.

Matthew had explained that he was going to work his way around the circle, pausing at each individual for a minute or two to concentrate on that person's problem. By the time he'd got half way around, I was ready to break the circle: I was in so much agony, I couldn't describe it to you. I didn't know whether I wanted to lie down, stand up, or bang my head against the wall – I was ready to quit. It was only the fact that the whole proceedings were being filmed that gave me the will power to remain where I was.

The moment he got to me and placed his left hand on my back and his right hand over the pain source, was the moment when the pain began to subside.

My wife, whose condition was unknown to Manning, and whom, I have to report, had suffered piteously with pain in the base of her neck – so much so that she hadn't slept or been able to rest properly for over eighteen months – also reported a reduction of her pain at that point.

By the time the proceedings were finished and we were down in the canteen enjoying a cup of coffee, the pain suffered by the pair of us had almost disappeared. In my wife's case, the condition has never returned.

Anyway, finally, I have to report that four months past my Royal Marsden die-by-date, I'm still fat, fit and hearty, still smoking, still getting pissed, still going to the dogs and enjoying life.

There have been many other instances of dramatic improvements in people after attending a circle. Mim Umney-Gray came to one of the healing circles I gave at the Rougemont Hotel in Exeter in June 1996 and wrote to me much later:

In around 1980 I had been prescribed glasses for reading and since then my eyesight had deteriorated to such an extent that by 1996 I was not only wearing glasses for reading, and the prescription was getting stronger and stronger, but I was also wearing contact lenses with glasses for driving and I was seeing less and less well. Night driving was becoming more and more difficult and as a result I was getting more and more depressed. I got to the stage that I felt as though I had permanent net curtains before my eyes. I was fifty-two and feeling pretty miserable about things.

After the first healing circle in June 1996 I started getting a very bad headache and by the time I left the hotel in the evening I did not know how I would drive home. On arriving home I went straight into the bathroom and removed my contact lenses. I will always remember it – it was a lovely summer's evening and as I walked into the garden to see my husband I discovered that I could see so vividly and clearly. Every stick of straw on the thatched roof of my neighbour's cottage stood out clearly and everywhere I looked was so incredibly clear and bright. I have never worn my contact lenses or spectacles since!

Also since then my long distance and middle distance sight is fine, clear and vivid. With regards to near sight I can now read without glasses and have indeed thrown them away.

After attending two healing circles in Bournemouth Mandy Player wrote to tell me that a cyst which she had had in her right breast for eleven years had started to 'dissolve'. Vicky Lee Millward also attended one of these circles in the hope that it would help a whiplash injury incurred in 1990 and a fracture to her arm sustained after falling down the stairs. She sent me a description of what happened:

After you came round and placed your hands on my shoulder, I experienced a terrible pain all down my right side. The pain felt like I was gripped in a vice. This pain lasted all through the session and left me when we opened our eyes.

Since the session I have been pain free, which is heaven.

The healing energy we send to others can be as potent as that which we generate on our own behalf. Pauline Allen of Eastleigh had attended a circle to help herself but had decided to think about a friend. In a letter to me she wrote:

> My friend has had cancer for five years and I have never seen her get out of her chair. I went through some amazing experiences in the healing circle. On my return home I was dying to see my friend but left it for two days. On seeing her, she looked wonderful . . . She couldn't understand the change in her feelings. Seeing her look so happy and pain free, I nearly cried. For over three weeks she ventured out of the house to meet friends. She was on a high.
>
> My friend was always negative about cancer and suppressed her feeling towards the disease. I gave her your tape, *Positive Approaches to Cancer*, and she was over the moon. This helped her understand a little more about how she was feeling and encouraged her to think positively.
>
> Sadly, Peggy died last week, but her family were so grateful that she had those few weeks pain-free and was able to go out of the house to meet her friends.

Lene Rønsholm sent healing energy to her mother during a demonstration I gave in front of over 1,000 people at the Concert House in Oslo. Her mother had been in hospital for ten weeks and because of lung damage was unable to breathe without the aid of a respirator. Two days before the demonstration the doctors at the hospital told Lene that it would be some time before her mother would be well enough to come off the respirator. When Lene visited the hospital the day after the circle she was told that her mother had breathed unassisted for four hours that day. A few days later her time off the respirator had increased to six hours.

Lene wrote: 'I don't know what's happening, but it is unbelievable . . . (No one will believe me when I tell them this, but I know your healing has something to do with it.)' My own belief is that Lene herself was responsible for guiding the energy to her mother.

It is almost impossible to tell who will benefit from healing. When I choose someone for a demonstration, I go purely on intuition – that little inner voice. The set-up with healing circles is different. I will give my energy to each person in the circle and rely on each of them to tune in as best they can. The energy generated by fifty or more people can be immensely powerful. Emotion pours out. Sometimes it is as though a wet flannel is being wrung out.

Some people derive instant benefit from this. Others are affected later and write to tell me that a long-standing problem has gone away. Workshops are different in format, with the emphasis on exercises that are designed to enhance people's healing abilities, but not in substance. Sometimes people will attend who seem unwilling to join in and I wonder what they will get out of it. However, I have learned that appearances can be very deceptive and just to experience the energy can be very beneficial. I received a very interesting letter after one workshop I gave in Cheshire.

> I came with my Mum and Dad. Dad is diabetic, suffers from glaucoma and is registered partially sighted. It was the very first time he had been to anything like your workshop and on the way to the car at the end of the session he said he had found it very interesting, although I know it had been difficult for him as he is very shy and feels embarrassed at being unable to stand for long.

> Anyway, twenty minutes later we hit the M56 motorway
> and suddenly he said, 'Goodness, I can see. I can see out
> of my bad eye. I can see the white van in front! I can see
> the red car!

At no point during the workshop had I touched Yvonne's father.
Yvonne, on the other hand, had spent the entire healing session
thinking hard about his eyes.

It is always gratifying to receive feedback, especially when it is
so positive. Yvonne wrote to me instantly to tell me of her father's
experience, as did Richard Stoakes. He had come to me for one-
to-one healing after a biopsy had confirmed a diagnosis of cancer
of the vocal chord. He then underwent a second biopsy for the
surgical 'stripping' of the site of the cancer. The Ear, Nose and
Throat specialist handling his case told him that radiotherapy
would be necessary if there were signs of further invasion after the
throat had settled from the biopsy. Richard came for his first
healing session in early September and had a second one a month
later. A few days after this second appointment, Richard faxed me:

> Last Tuesday when I saw you, I told you that I felt some-
> thing happening in my throat during the session and that
> when I concentrated something in my head seemed to
> be 'in tune'.
>
> Once I was in the car on the way to pick up the family
> in Bury St Edmunds I tried my voice – amazing! Pavarotti
> won't have sleepless nights yet but what a difference!
>
> When I got back I tried it out on the family and they
> were speechless, which makes a change for them. Now I
> can order a pint in a pub without being ignored.

Richard went back to the hospital for a check-up after this second
session. His ENT specialist described as 'quite remarkable' the
speed and degree of healing that had taken place in his throat.
Richard has continued having healing regularly – 'just in case the
Phantom of the Opera croaks and gets stuck in the chandelier'.

Even now, on each visit, he notices the effect the healing has on his voice insofar as altering its pitch and timbre. At the end of 1998 he was having six-monthly check-ups with his specialist.

* * *

The summer of 1996 was an eventful one. Henrietta voted with her feet and decided that she wanted to live with Gig and me at Sturgeon's Hall. Christine's drinking had long been a source of friction, as had the constant stream of invective against Gig and myself. I hoped this would lessen over time but it seemed to be getting worse.

Also that summer I received an unexpected call from Paradine, asking me to contribute to a third *Beyond Belief*. Despite reservations, I convinced myself that it would be better this time. The executive whose attitude had so riled me had left Carlton to do his worst elsewhere and the word 'interactive' was not uttered. However, apart from a couple of amazing telepathy experiments involving Uri, the programme was a damp squib. If it had not been for a recent experience with Gig, it would have been even worse from my perspective.

Gig had been given three rings by her mother, one circled with diamonds, the second circled with rubies and the third circled with emeralds. Although immensely pleased with her gifts, Gig was unsure how to wear them because they were a bit tight. One Sunday evening she was experimenting and put all three rings on one finger. All three got stuck. She pulled and pulled, but to no avail. I suggested that we leave them until the morning and then try again.

We went to bed and had not been lying there for longer than a few minutes when Gig started to panic. Her finger felt very painful and she was convinced it was swelling up. If it was not swollen at this point, it quickly became so. We tried everything we could think of to prise off the rings, starting with washing-up liquid and soap. Then I got some iced water, which I hoped would reduce the swelling. Gig put her hand into the water but soon withdrew it because of the severe pain it caused her. Eventually we admitted defeat and went to the casualty department of the local hospital, where the rings were eased off with the assistance of KY jelly.

This experience gave me an idea for *Beyond Belief 3*, to demonstrate the effectiveness of healing in controlling pain. For the show we filled a large glass tank with iced water and invited *Sunday Times* columnist Hazel Courtney to be my guinea pig. I asked Hazel to place one hand in the water and see how long she could keep it there. She managed twenty-five seconds before an intense burning sensation forced her to withdraw it.

A few minutes later she put her other hand in the tank, while I gave her healing. Her experience this time was quite different. After fifty-eight seconds she could still not feel the effects of the cold. Her awareness was of heat coming down her arm and into her hand. Dr Brian Roet was on hand to explain. In the first part of the experiment the effect of the cold on the blood vessels had caused a message to be sent to the brain, registering pain. The healing had blocked the pain pathway, preventing the brain registering the pain.

My inability to come up with another 'first' for the show left me open to a suggestion by David which I was reluctant to take up. He wanted me to revisit our interview of 1974 and 'do' a couple of Thomas Penn diagnoses. I had said goodbye to Thomas Penn for the best of reasons and it seemed wrong to reintroduce him just because I could not devise an alternative that would convince David. However, that was what happened, and I took a step backwards momentarily. I paid the price. Both diagnoses fell flat, although I sensed that one of them was accurate and the person concerned was not telling the truth.

I was an awestruck bystander for what was undoubtedly the most memorable aspect of that final *Beyond Belief*. Uri's coup for the show had been to persuade former CIA officer Major David Morehouse to take part in an experiment involving what is called 'remote viewing'. Morehouse had previously been employed by the US military to teach service personnel how to perfect this technique, which had been used to try and discern the layouts of sensitive enemy targets, such as nuclear submarines and military installations.

The original plan was for Morehouse, who was in a TV studio in Washington, to choose from five sealed envelopes handed to him on air, each of them containing instructions on how to reach a particular building or landmark in Washington, and for Uri to telepathically guide Morehouse to the destination given in the chosen envelope.

This rather elaborate exercise had to be abandoned at the last minute when a blizzard in Washington forced Morehouse to stay inside the studio building. It was decided that a photograph of each building or landmark would be substituted for the set of instructions in the envelopes. Morehouse opened the envelope, looked at the image and then transmitted its identity to Uri, who then had to draw it. At no point during this exercise could Morehouse see Uri or Uri see the image Morehouse was looking at. Within thirty seconds Uri had drawn the image, and got it absolutely right.

The speed with which he read the information coming to him from Morehouse gave the production team a major problem. Four minutes had been allowed in the schedule for this particular exercise and now they had three and a half minutes with nothing to fill them. Uri came spontaneously to the rescue. Elated by his success, he was keen to capitalize on it and prove it had not been a fluke. He turned to one of the floor managers and said, 'Quick, get me something, anything!'

This man had a bottle of water at the ready in case anybody wanted a drink. He handed Uri the bottle. Uri now said to David Morehouse over the transatlantic link, 'I am now looking at something. I am going to project it to you. You draw what I am looking at.' Within a very short space of time Morehouse had drawn the bottle. This was amazing enough but it was not half as amazing as the discovery we made after the show.

A couple of hours before the programme had been due to go on air, Morehouse had arrived at the Washington studio and said to the production team, 'They are going to try and pull a fast one on me.' Nothing was further from our minds, so how he got this idea is a mystery – the show was risky enough without asking for trouble. Anyway, he had asked for a piece of paper and a pen and had made a drawing – of a bottle. Incredibly, somehow he had picked up Uri's spontaneous 'flash' hours before it had occurred.

I would have felt worse about that last *Beyond Belief* if I had received no indication that it had done some good. A retired nurse, Anne Penman, wrote on 23 February, the day after the show was broadcast:

> ### Dear Mr Manning
>
> I was born on 7th March 1919 and have had several damaged discs and a chipped vertebra. At the age of ten I was told that I would never see forty as my heart and kidneys were damaged as a result of diphtheria. Nevertheless I have arrived into old age.
>
> Now comes the 'Beyond Belief' part, for somehow I had tapped into healing heat which covered the kidney area of my back, then descended to ease the pain of an injury I received early in 1940, which makes sitting a problem. For the first time in fifty-seven years I was pain-free!
>
> I do not know if the relief will be permanent, but I must thank you very sincerely for a very pleasurable experience.

Letters like this convince me that, for all its shortcomings, *Beyond Belief* did not succeed in trivializing what I do. The awareness it raised in the majority may have been temporary, but if there is a significant minority in whom the idea of healing remains, the experience will have been worthwhile. Fundamentally, people *know* what is true and what is not, and if something strikes a chord in them they will accept it, even though they may not be able to give a rational explanation.

Coincidentally, or perhaps not, Susanna Lee of Oxford also put pen to paper on the same day as Anne Penman:

Dear Matthew

One year ago today I participated in your healing circle in Kensington. I remember you saying how much you'd welcome any feedback and I have been meaning to write for some time.

I had been trying to have a baby for five and a half years. Medically, apparently, there was nothing wrong with either myself or my husband but still nothing happened. I had almost given up hope. A friend suggested I went to one of your circles.

During the course of the hour we sat linked together, I had many thoughts. I worked quite hard at constructing positive mental images of people I knew who were ill, whereas an astonishingly clear picture of myself with a fully pregnant belly and one even more clear of a wicker cot on which holly leaves were attached just spontaneously came to mind with no effort on my part. My husband is half Chinese but has little contact with his family on that side. I found myself conversing with his grandfather who had long since died and saying how much I wanted to extend the 'Lee' family.

After the session I went to buy bread in a department store. The cashier was Chinese. I signed a cheque with my married name 'Lee'. The cashier commented that that was his name too. When I said that mine was also from China, he held the queue up and wrote the Chinese characters on the back of the till receipt saying that the 'Lee's' were a very big family.

Two weeks later I was pregnant. I hardly dared to bring myself to write to you because I couldn't believe my luck. On 23rd November, exactly nine months after that day in Kensington, our little girl was born. She is absolute heaven and I am totally convinced that this is as a result of your circle.

For this gift I cannot possibly convey enough thanks. To my mind it is also an extraordinary string of events which

can be added to what must be a vast collection of similar
such anecdotes from people who have had the benefit
of your healing.

* * *

In the autumn of 1997 I received a letter from Earl Baldwin of
Bewdley, Chairman of the Parliamentary Group for Alternative
and Complementary Medicine, who asked if I would be prepared
to talk to this group about healing. The group had been set up
in order to try and give legal status to the various different complementary therapies. Thanks in no small measure to the
enthusiasm of the group's treasurer, Conservative MP David
Tredinnick, it had succeeded in getting such protection for
acupuncture and osteopathy and was now looking to extend it
to include other complementary therapies, including healing.

Harry Edwards was responsible for getting healing decrimi-
nalized in Great Britain, but I was aware from first-hand
experience of its criminal status in many other European countries. Tredinnick told me that moves were afoot in Brussels to
set European standards by which complementary therapists
would be subject to the same codes of conduct and discipline as
other medical practitioners. This is a good idea. At the moment
in Britain, anybody can set themselves up as a complementary
therapist, and too many people do so with very slender credentials. This is clearly wrong and it must be possible to devise some
form of recognized evaluation to protect the general public
against the unscrupulous or the incompetent.

However, the situation with healing is more complex and of
all the complementary therapies it would be the most difficult
to assess by means of a set of formal criteria. I have no medical
knowledge, nor do I need it in the way I work. I am not making
diagnoses, nor do I prescribe powerful substances as remedies.
I will not accept patients unless they have been diagnosed by a
qualified doctor. As to assessing my competence – how could
this be done? In the end, the proof is in the eating – if people feel

that it benefits them and their symptoms are alleviated by its use, then it has to be said to be of value, even though no scientific yardstick yet exists which can explain the how.

Gig and I went to the Houses of Parliament on 28 October, during a gap in the schedule of my British tour. It was quite an experience. The committee room was packed with a wide cross-section of people involved in complementary medicine, as well as MPs who had not previously attended the group's meetings.

After explaining my work I decided to raise the temperature by telling them about the antagonism towards healing shown by the German authorities. I had been at the receiving end of another dose of this relatively recently, in 1995, when Walter had organized an evening healing demonstration and a weekend workshop in Berlin. He had felt that Berlin was far enough away from the places where we had encountered problems previously. Neither of us had bargained on my name being on some list of undesirables.

As soon as I had presented my passport on arrival in Berlin, it had been held. Gig and I had stood there for ten minutes while officials had cross-checked information and tapped it into a computer. They had allowed us entry, but presumably only so that the relevant authority could be alerted to deal with me. We had reached the venue to find the police ready with a threat supported by the relevant paperwork: if I gave a healing demonstration, I would be arrested and the promoter would be fined £20,000. Needless to say, we had not doubted that they would keep their word.

In the letter of thanks David Tredinnick sent to me a few days after my talk to the parliamentary group, I was pleased to note that he seemed to have taken my concern seriously: 'Your experiences in Germany gave a stark warning of the threat to healing in this country, which we must address in Parliament, perhaps at some stage in the near future. Certainly it is essential for us to be vigilant concerning all European legislation and Directives.'

* * *

In a book called *Vibrational Medicine*, Richard Gerber describes the beneficial effects that 'healed' water can have on living things, from plants to human beings. According to the experimental work done by Dr Bernard Grad of Montreal's McGill University in the 1960s – which was later supported by the work of research chemist Dr Robert Miller – water undergoes a physical change when it is healed, with a shift in the bond angle of the molecule. The significant reduction in surface tension that is evident in 'healed' water is similar to the effect seen in water exposed to magnetic fields.

Further experiments demonstrated that the energy stored in such treated water releases gradually over a twenty-four-hour period, at the end of which the surface tension returns to normal. A rapid discharge of energy could be effected if a metallic rod touched the charged water or if the charged water was poured into a stainless steel container. Metal could also be used to direct the energy to where it might be needed. The first healer to believe that energized water could benefit the sick was Franz Anton Mesmer in the eighteenth century. In his treatments he used a method called a 'bacquet', in which several bottles of 'healed' water were connected to patients via metal rods.

I was curious to see whether the benefits of healing might not be extended by using this principle. I asked people attending my circles to bring a bottle of water with them and place it between their feet or under their seat. It soon became evident that the energy going around the circle infused the water, producing incredible effects when the 'healed' liquid was subsequently drunk. One girl who came to three circles I gave in Scotland had what she identified as an hallucinogenic experience after drinking a litre of 'healed' water one evening. Gig had a similar experience while sipping 'healed' water and reading a copy of *The Link* a day or two after our first meeting, when the room filled with amazing colours.

I am always looking for ways of prolonging the good effect of healing. The use of 'healed' water is one way, music another. Music makes a huge difference to the healing experience, softening the atmosphere and enhancing people's receptivity. It dissipates the hard, cold edge of silence and aids relaxation. I deliberately choose descriptive music that I hope will conjure up visual images and quite literally transport people to the furthest reaches of their imagination. I am always pushing the limits to see what I can get away with.

I tend to use music that other healers would probably think inappropriate. I have never subscribed to the idea that music for healing should be pretty and emotionally bland. Music that lifts us and makes us want to fly, in our hearts and minds, does far more by way of engendering a positive outlook. Passivity is the last attitude to be encouraged, especially with cancer patients. They need strength to win the fight and music can represent energy and grit as well as inspire hope.

The purpose of using music in my work is to fix an association with the healing experience and enable people to revisit that experience whenever they choose. Many of my patients – and the people who come to my healing circles – will ask me for details of the music I have been playing and will subsequently buy a copy of the disc to enable them to play it at home. In this way they are able to prolong the benefits of healing by linking the music they hear during healing with the act itself.

In some cases this connection is very intense and people can receive vivid imagery, they can sense changes occurring and also feel the heat of my hands. I am always careful to use music that people are very unlikely to have heard in another connection, because a piece of music, like a perfume, can have very powerful emotions attached to it. There are many well-known compositions that I find uplifting and positive, but I will not use them because there is no guarantee they will not arouse some painful memory in others.

Years ago I was working with a woman who had cancer. She had a cassette tape of relaxation music that included many well-known pieces of classical music played on the harp and flute. She carried this tape with her everywhere, and even when she was undergoing chemotherapy in hospital she would listen to it.

Almost a year later she was watching television one night when an advertisement for a particular brand of paint was shown. Suddenly, she felt very nauseous and ran to the bathroom because she thought she was going to be sick. This feeling passed very quickly and she felt fine again.

She could not understand what had happened. Later the same week the same advertisement came on while she was watching television, and again she felt very sick. Then she remembered: the background music used in the commercial was one of the pieces on the cassette tape she had used during her illness. She realizes that she will never be able to listen to this piece of music again without her body associating it with her experience of illness.

I should have remembered this lesson when I treated orchestral conductor Arthur Davison, although his aversion to the familiar turned out to be for a different reason. Charming and courteous though he was, I was a bit intimidated by having to select music for someone with his professional background. Somehow it did not seem appropriate to select one of my usual companions, Kitaro, Vangelis or Tim Wheater.

I chose a tape from the small amount of classical recordings in my collection and began the session. After about a minute he turned to me and said: 'I don't know whether you put this music on for your benefit or mine, but if you've got it on for my benefit I don't find it relaxing at all. I'm sitting here counting in all the instruments. Have you got any good modern jazz?' I had not, and he discovered Kitaro and Tim Wheater instead.

Linda McGinley's husband has never been a patient of mine. His wife started coming to me in early 1998 for a form of neuralgia that had given her severe pains across her face and in the back of her head for almost nineteen years. In recent years the pain had got worse and despite seeing numerous doctors and having blood tests, brain scans, an EEG, and being checked from head to toe many times, nobody could find the cause of the pain. She had taken all sorts of medicine, both conventional and complementary, but none had alleviated the problem. She was now desperate, and wrote: 'Please, please can you help me as this pain seems to control my life and prevent me from doing many things I would like to do.'

After a few months of receiving healing, Linda was feeling much better. She was working on herself at home, too, allowing time for creative visualization and meditation using a tape of Kitaro's music.

Linda's husband suffered from a potentially crippling disease called ankylosing spondylitis, in which vertebrae in the spine fuse together, severely limiting movement. Early one morning he was woken by a terrible pain in his back and chest. Desperate for relief, he put on the Kitaro tape, got back into bed and started thinking about me, repeating my name and asking for my help. After a while he suddenly felt an intense heat burning him. This sensation became so intense that he shot out of bed, certain that he must have dropped a lighted cigarette among the bedclothes. Once he was up he realized the pain had gone. It has not returned.

Eric Clapton once said that his ideal would be to go on stage, strike one chord and have the whole audience in a state of ecstasy. When I am healing, I aim to get the person to the highest level of receptivity on one wave of energy. Music undoubtedly helps this process of transcendence and is perhaps one of the purest means by which it can be achieved. In my experience, Kitaro is the musician who has come closest to achieving Clapton's ideal.

I discovered Kitaro's music during a trip to the States in the early 1980s. I began to use it during healing, alongside that of Vangelis, another musician whose work gives off an amazing, positive energy. Kitaro's compositions embody a desire to connect old and new and to reveal the interdependence of humanity and nature. Kitaro himself spends a lot of his time touring, drawing inspiration from the diversity of world cultures and then feeding back his impressions and experiences to listeners. He has said, 'Feeling is the most important element in my music,' and certainly warmth and emotion transcend the undoubtedly brilliant technical underpinnings.

Gig and I got to meet Kitaro in March 1998 in Amsterdam, which was the last stop on his European tour for the year. London had almost happened until a problem with getting the musicians' equipment to the Barbican Hall in time had proved insuperable. I am sure he would have attracted a large audience in Britain and probably I would have seen a number of familiar faces. When his music was finally released in Britain his recording company had put a prepaid reply slip inside each CD asking people to say how they had come to hear of Kitaro. According to the record company, 90 per cent of respondents put my name on the slip.

As a performer and as himself Kitaro inhabits an ego-free zone. On stage he stands in profile to the audience with his keyboards sideways on to the audience. The members of his band are similarly retiring and hug the edges of the performing space. It is all very un-rock and a wonderful example of someone getting very close to sublimating his ego. In Amsterdam we in the audience were aware solely of the music communicating with the spirit, embracing us and drawing us into a communion of equals. Some of it makes you feel like getting up and dancing. But no one ever dances at a Kitaro concert. Many people cry, but no one dances.

Kitaro did not say a word until the very end, when he thanked us all for coming. There was a long queue of people wanting to speak to him afterwards. Gig and I went backstage and waited alongside them while he completed the twenty minutes or so he takes for meditation after each show. Kitaro very rarely gives interviews to journalists. His treatment of admirers is another matter. He will spend hours talking to them and never begrudges them his time. The previous night, in Brussels, 300 people had been waiting to speak to him and he had sat there until the last person had gone home. Kitaro was a revelation to us. A man with loving, sparkling eyes who creates sounds that make the soul dance.

Chapter 7

CHIRON'S CHALLENGE

Experiencing Kitaro live was like suddenly finding oneself in bright sunlight after a spell in too-cool shadow. I had been relieved to see the back of 1997 and hopeful that 1998 would restore my zest and enthusiasm. The final third of the year had been the worst, coinciding with a thirty-date British tour of healing circles and workshops. I had strangely mixed feelings about this tour without knowing why. These feelings had nothing to do with the tour itself or the people I met, although I did get very fed up staying in bad hotels; I have never understood why it is that the standards in British hotels and restaurants generally are so abysmal in comparison with elsewhere in the world and the prices so high.

I felt very unsettled and caught myself wondering 'Why am I doing this?' I concluded that I must be suffering from burn-out as a consequence of working relentlessly for some twenty years with few breaks. It was not surprising I was getting tired of saying and doing the same things. I addressed the perceived problem by deciding not to tour in 1998, except for one brief trip to Norway, and to spend the year at home, thinking about my life and through this process finding alternative ways of presenting healing. With my immediate future now settled, I expected to feel more relaxed, but the uneasiness persisted.

On New Year's Eve both Gig and I were hit by very strange emotions. Gig was very prickly and not at all her usual easy-going self. I felt as though I was being mentally attacked by something horribly black and negative. This nasty sensation did not pass entirely. No amount of rationalizing would push away its residue, although sometimes I would be less aware of it. On 2 May 1998, I was not aware of it at all. That was the day Gig and I got married.

Some people expressed surprise that we should bother, but it had always been our intention to marry once my divorce came through. The knowledge that a piece of paper would not alter the shape of our life together made no difference. We wanted to make our union complete by going through a public ritual witnessed by those dearest to us – sixteen people in all, twelve family and four close friends.

That wonderful day began unpromisingly with grey skies and high winds. We brightened it up at around 8.30 a.m. by opening our first bottle of vintage champagne. A second bottle was awaiting us in the white stretch limousine loaned by friends to take us to the registry office in Bury St Edmunds. As we glided through the lanes, sipping our champagne and enjoying the glorious views splashed with the yellow of the rape seed fields, the clouds parted and the sun beamed down. It seemed a very fitting salutation.

✳   ✳   ✳

After our wedding life went on very much as before, except that Gig had to get used to having a new surname. It was lovely to be able to spend so much more time at home. My environment has always been enormously important to me and one of the reasons why I was so unhappy at Sturgeon's Hall before Gig came along was that I was living in a house that seemed to be reflecting back my unhappiness. And yet I knew it was the right house. When I was about eight or nine years old I had a map of Suffolk on which I drew a triangle. I promised myself that when I was older I would live within this triangle. Sturgeon's Hall is situated right in the middle of it.

I like my father's philosophy when it comes to property. He says that we may think we own buildings but we are only ever their custodians. This makes perfect sense when you consider that the life of a house is usually very much longer than our own, and that the energy within it changes with each new set of occupants.

Sturgeon's Hall was in a very poor state when I bought it in 1990. It had been lived in but neglected. There were broken windows with balls of newspaper stuffed into the holes to keep out the elements. Plants were growing through the floor. A wall at the front of the house had rotted through at ground level and was flapping in the wind. The kitchen was in such a disgusting state I had to hire industrial cleaners to remove the thick grease that coated every surface.

When I started pulling the place apart, I discovered its medieval origins. I restored these wherever possible and undid the Victorianization of the roof spaces by returning them to their original vaulted state. However, all I had done before Gig moved in was to renovate the shell. It has taken our joint energy and enthusiasm to create the look and feel of the house and garden as they are today. Gig's mother has a fabulous garden in Gloucestershire and so from a very early age Gig has been aware of gardening as a creative activity. I have always liked gardens but not until we began to plan the garden at Sturgeon's Hall did I appreciate the deep satisfaction that tending plants can give.

The similarities between gardening and healing seemed very apparent in the growing season that year. I did not know when I bought Sturgeon's Hall that a ley line runs right through the room I use for healing and into part of the garden where there is a gazebo. The plants closest to the ley line seem to do spectacularly well in terms of their height and vigour. We had daffodils planted in a bed outside the window of the healing room which grew to almost four feet in the spring. Later in the year the daisies by the gazebo reached over eight feet.

*   *   *

In July 1998 Gig and I discovered the cause of the oppressive 'cloud' that seemed to be shadowing us.

Around the turn of the year Gig had developed what she thought were haemorrhoids and had started going to different complementary therapists for treatment. I had been a bit sceptical about the wisdom of this without a diagnosis. I am all for alternatives so long as they are proven alternatives and the practitioners know what they are dealing with. None of the remedies she tried was successful in clearing up the problem and she began to develop worrying and distressing symptoms, including acute pain. Clearly, something was wrong.

Gig found a GP from whom she would be happy to take advice. Perhaps it was because his father had been a homeopath, but this man exuded a personal quality that encouraged trust. He took one look and diagnosed thrombotic haemorrhoids, which he thought would probably have to be removed surgically. Within three days Gig was referred to a consultant in Bury St Edmunds who took a biopsy because he was not sure they were haemorrhoids. He found a lump which further investigation identified as malignant.

I had spent the best part of twenty years working with people with cancer, but this did not prepare me for the bombshell that hit me when the diagnosis was given. I could not think straight. My brain seemed to be in paralysis. I cancelled my appointments for the week. It would have been dishonourable for me to continue working with my patients when I was incapable of focusing properly.

It was then arranged that Gig and I should see an oncologist from Addenbrookes Hospital in Cambridge, which is reputedly one of the best hospitals in the country outside London. The oncologist was a woman in her late thirties. I have listened for years to my patients' complaints about the lack of communication skills among doctors. This woman had none whatsoever. Furthermore, she made no attempt to disguise the fact. On the rare occasions she made eye contact, it was always with me. Mostly, though, she directed her gaze away from us. This was not a promising beginning and as she spoke the scenario got worse. She launched into treatment proposals.

We wanted to know what might have caused the cancer. She said she did not know. It was a rare cancer; only 300 people a year in Britain are diagnosed with it, 200 of whom are over the age of 70. In a handful of cases in men, it was AIDS related. This piece of information was tossed off almost as an aside. At this point Gig started panicking. The oncologist was oblivious to her reaction and ploughed on with her proposal.

The treatment would have to be carried out at Addenbrookes, and would involve chemotherapy and radiotherapy followed by a radioactive implant. Both Gig and I had taken an instant dislike to the oncologist, and her description of the treatment did not make us feel any better disposed towards her. If we were to follow the route she was suggesting, it would have to be with someone we could relate to and who acknowledged our anxieties and feelings. At this early stage, however, we could not accept this as our sole option. We wanted to discover what, if any, alternatives were available.

One of my patients had told me about a clinic in southern Germany where the treatment was based on the principle that cancerous tumours do not like changes in temperature, so if the temperature in surrounding tissue can be either raised or lowered the tumour will tend to die back. We wanted to visit this clinic before we made a decision on which form of treatment to accept. The oncologist from Addenbrookes was very sceptical and told us that the type of therapy we were describing was not radical and had been known about since the eighteenth century. I asked her if it would be safe to leave our decision for two or three weeks. She said she would be just about happy to delay treatment that long, but no longer.

The following day she telephoned me at home and told me that it would not matter where we went in the world or who we saw, they would in the end suggest the treatment she was offering. She then tried to pressurize me into getting Gig to accept her proposal.

A couple of days later we flew out to the clinic in southern Germany. Our hopes were high. We had received a good report

of the place and by this route Gig would avoid chemotherapy
and radiotherapy. We realized soon after arrival that this was not
the answer. The atmosphere was hard, and so was the treatment.

In one type of therapy the patient is placed in what looks
like a perspex coffin and is then subjected to the temperature
inside this structure being raised to as high a point as the person
can take without expiring. The two doctors who ran the place
wanted to use 'galvo' treatment on Gig's tumour. This would
involve passing an electrical current into the tumour via a very
fine wire. One of the doctors assured us of its effectiveness and
said the tumour would be gone after ten days. I did not trust
him or this claim.

As we waited in reception shortly before our departure, I
struck up conversation with an American doctor who had come
over to look at the clinic with a view to sending some of his
patients there. I told him about our situation and asked him what
would happen if Gig went through with the heat and 'galvo'
treatments. In his opinion the tumour might disappear temporarily, but the treatments were stop-gaps and not cures.

When we got back to England we received individual proposals from the two doctors at the clinic. I thought it was rather
disturbing that two no doubt highly qualified specialists working
together out of the same clinic should send us different treatment plans. Both Gig and I felt very low at this point, because we
had thought that clinic would provide the answer.

Gig would have been happy to have allowed me to give her
healing and not to have had medical treatment. However, I was
not prepared to take that responsibility. We were luckier than
most couples in that, by virtue of my work and contacts, I was
well positioned to run to earth the people who could advise us
on the various options. It would then be for Gig to decide on the
treatment she wanted.

Among the stack of books and articles in my office was information on both alternative and orthodox treatments for cancer,
all of them seemingly mutually exclusive. Everybody seemed to
have their own particular belief system, axe to grind or product

to sell. I felt as though we were in a bazaar surrounded by rival traders and soothsayers. I was acutely conscious of the passing days as we sifted and considered. If the first oncologist was to be believed, time was a luxury we did not have.

I suggested to Gig that we should try to get an appointment with Professor Karol Sikora, the one person I would go to if I were to develop cancer. Gig had been introduced to his approach through a book he had co-authored with Dr Hilary Thomas, called *A Positive Approach to Cancer*, which set out the various treatments clearly, sensibly and sensitively.

I had first come across Karol Sikora in the late Eighties when I had given a talk to medical students at the Hammersmith Hospital. I had been favourably impressed by his relaxed manner and his receptiveness to different ideas. More recently Sikora had been seconded to the World Health Organization, where he was chief of their cancer programme, and was only working part time at the Hammersmith. Gig was very fortunate to get an appointment within three days of our GP writing to him and mentioning my name. This was a significant turning point.

After looking at the CAT scans and examining Gig, Sikora advised us not to rush into any form of treatment. He thought the tumour might be operable, which from Gig's perspective would be a kinder option than chemotherapy and radiotherapy. I asked him the same question I had put to the first oncologist: why had this happened? He did not know. It was such an unusual cancer, especially in someone of Gig's age, that he could not draw any conclusions from it. He estimated that the tumour had been in situ for up to five years. In his opinion, though, if anyone has to have cancer, this particular tumour was the best kind to have, because it is very slow growing and tends not to spread. He advised us to talk to the surgeon before making a decision. There was no rush. Nothing untoward would happen with the cancer while we were making up our minds. His words came as a great relief. I had not said as much to Gig, but I had been desperately worried that the cancer might have gone into other organs.

I cannot over-emphasize the difference between our conversation with Sikora and the one we had had with the oncologist from Addenbrookes. Both doctors are cancer specialists so their depth of knowledge of the disease must be comparable, and yet one could be forgiven for thinking they were considering different cases. The Addenbrookes oncologist could have given us the news that anyone who is told they have cancer must surely want to hear – it is a very slow-growing kind and tends not to produce secondaries. She had needlessly given us the impression that the prognosis was gloomy when the reality was that it was about as positive as a diagnosis of cancer can be. No doubt she is brilliant on the technical aspects of her specialism, but medicine is about much more than being a technician. The best doctors are also healers, and their reasons for being drawn into medicine in the first place are bound up with this innate ability.

We went to see the colorectal surgeon with our hopes high that Gig would be able to avoid chemotherapy and radiotherapy. We were to be disappointed. In his opinion surgery was not the solution, unless Gig was prepared to have a permanent colostomy. She was not and we came away feeling deflated. Sikora's optimism had been contagious. We discovered at this point how thin the line is between being unrealistically positive and realistically positive.

However, it would not be fair to blame Sikora for this. I had a great deal to thank him for. He was responsible for putting me back on the tracks after shock and anxiety had temporarily thrown me off them. I had done so much work with cancer patients that I knew too much in one sense, and too little in another. Information poured into us from all sides, from patients and friends wanting to help. Shortly after Gig had been diagnosed, I was given some figures on anal cancers which had come off the Internet and these gave a life expectancy of seventeen months.

I was devastated. Common sense should have reminded me that such statistics are unhelpful and do not differentiate between types of tumour and their behaviour patterns. There are about

200 kinds of cancer, all of them different. Like most people for whom cancer becomes a reality, the word does not reflect such distinctions, so one goes through a nightmare phase of being prey to one's worst fears. Once Gig decided to opt for treatment at the Hammersmith, I threw out most of that material.

We were told that the proposed treatment would last seven weeks. The first stage of the treatment would involve chemotherapy in weeks one and five and radiotherapy every day for five weeks. There would then be a break of two weeks, followed by two further weeks of radiotherapy. One of the consultant oncologists handling Gig's treatment, Dr Pat Price, told us that the tumour would in all probability still be detectable at the end of the treatment. Radiotherapy works over a long period and takes time to break down malignancy.

Both of us feared that the chemotherapy would have unpleasant side-effects and assumed that Gig would lose her hair as a matter of course. Thankfully the drug she was given – 5FU – did not cause this to happen, and there are other forms of chemotherapy that do not either. In addition to the conventional treatment, Gig took full advantage of the complementary therapies on offer at the hospital, especially reflexology, which she found very effective in helping her to relax. On her own initiative she had already contacted the Bristol Cancer Care Centre for advice on vitamin and mineral therapy. One of my patients passed on a vital piece of knowledge concerning a product called Bromaline, a pineapple extract whose positive benefits in the treatment of cancer – especially in conjunction with the drug 5FU – have been reported in over 200 medical journals around the world.

We had not gone to Karol Sikora just because he is, in my opinion, the top oncologist in Britain, but because of his approach to cancer. It was no accident that I had given a talk to those students at the Hammersmith. Sikora is known to be sympathetic to complementary therapies and has been influenced by the work of the Bristol Cancer Help Centre, where people are encouraged to fight cancer with a combination of treatments,

conventional and complementary, including healing, diet, counselling and stress control.

He has been quoted as saying that 'a little bit of Bristol makes
my medicine go down', and has been instrumental in developing formal links with the Centre so that patients in his unit at
Hammersmith can benefit from the expertise on offer in Bristol.
Sikora's attitude is exceptional among top British oncologists,
some of whom are hostile to any treatment that is not strictly
orthodox.

One of my patients who was receiving treatment at another
hospital had the misfortune to discover just how vehement was
her consultant's dislike of anything 'alternative'. She had a book
by Penny Brohn, one of the founders of the Bristol Cancer Help
Centre, on her bedside table in the hospital. When he saw it, he
picked it up and said 'You shouldn't be reading this kind of
rubbish!', then threw it across the room. If his behaviour is any
indicator, there is still a long way to go before the medical profession as a whole accepts the validity of multiple approaches to
cancer.

However, as Gig and I have discovered, the Hammersmith
Hospital is an oasis of hope and progressive thinking. The Cancer
Centre has a full-time complementary therapies coordinator and it
is possible to receive – on the National Health Service, alongside
conventional medical treatment – reflexology, massage and aro-
matherapy. They are looking to improve their provision by offering
additional complementary therapies in the future. I was thrilled to
see advertisements for my cassettes. As Professor Sikora has said:
'The whole shift now is towards the total care of cancer patients.'

This was just the approach Gig was looking for. The whole
team at the Hammersmith Cancer Unit is dedicated to putting
patients first. This means answering any questions fully yet com-
passionately, providing reassurance and support when it is
necessary and generally creating an atmosphere in which patients
feel relaxed and confident. It is impossible to underestimate the
importance to cancer patients of being treated by people who
understand their needs and are prepared to meet them.

My experience has convinced me that this approach works, and it is one that many people naturally lean towards. Some of my patients have succeeded in devising their own versions of Bristol.

Carol Downham was in her early fifties when she was diagnosed with a rare cancer of the womb. She had a hysterectomy and was told that the chances of the cancer returning were 'practically nil'. In July 1995 she began to suffer from abdominal pains which her doctor put down to irritable bowel syndrome. Three months later she was rushed into hospital with suspected appendicitis.

When the surgeon opened her up he discovered malignancy in the bowel and peritoneum. He removed as much as he could, but in January 1996 the cancer flared up again, this time between her intestines and bladder. She was then referred to the Royal Marsden where chemotherapy was the suggested treatment. She refused this and went to a homeopath, who put her on vitamins and antioxidants. In March 1996 she began a course of chemotherapy at Addenbrookes Hospital in Cambridge, which gave partially encouraging results – a CAT scan in July revealing the lumps had gone although the 'cancer cells were still there'. On 25 July she was rushed back into hospital after developing a high temperature, and given antibiotics.

Carol had been carrying my address and telephone number around in her purse for three months before she finally got down to writing to me. She had switched on the television one evening, seen me and taken this as an omen that she should get in touch. I was unable to see Carol on a one-to-one basis before 11 September and my assistants suggested that she attend a healing circle I was to give in Cambridge on 31 July.

Carol was still in hospital undergoing antibiotic therapy, but she insisted on being allowed out so that she could come to the circle. The hospital staff were used to her rather irregular ways – enjoying the occasional cigarette in the hospital bathroom or, on chemotherapy days, to avoid the hated institutional food, reserving her bed in the morning and then telling the shocked staff that she would be back later in good time to receive her treatment.

In December 1996 Carol's oncologist wrote to her, confirming the results of a Magnetic Resonance Imaging scan and a separate chest X-ray. There was 'no sign of secondaries in the lungs and, as I told you on the telephone, the MR confirms the absence of anything sinister in liver, kidneys, spleen or para-aortic lympth nodes'.

Carol is still coming for healing every other month. She is also still taking homeopathic remedies, receiving reflexology when she feels the need and using creative visualization and relaxation techniques. In other words, she is doing everything that she considers necessary to keep her well and free from stress – the cause, she believes, of her health problems, which developed after a particularly painful divorce in 1990, initially with high blood pressure requiring medication, and shingles.

Sue Wallis is another of my natural 'battlers' who has cherry-picked from the help and information available to pull herself through. In January 1994 she was diagnosed with cancer of the lining of the lung, for which, she was told, there was no treatment apart from radiotherapy to reduce the swelling. The radiotherapy was palliative, to make Sue more comfortable and ease her principal symptom of shortness of breath. Asked how long she could expect to live, her consultant told her that it would be a 'miracle' if she was still alive in twelve months. She said, 'I believe in miracles – you can help me make one happen.'

Sue told me that her overriding feeling – after she and her husband had got over the initial shock and fear – was of being cheated. She was forty-two, happily married with a sixteen-year-old daughter and had just finished a five-year course in a subject she loved. The future had looked so bright and promising.

Sue decided to fight and direct her anger at the cells that had 'gone wrong'. Someone gave her my tape *Fighting Back* and she started using the self-healing techniques straight away.

> I'm sure it was Matthew's voice that got me through those
> initial traumatic days and weeks. I loved doing the tape.
> It enabled me to create a profoundly peaceful space, a
> quietness in all the madness that had become my life. At
> first I did it two or three times every day. I imagined pure
> white dogs with white eyes, sleek and strong, bounding
> through my body – hundreds and thousands of them
> searching for anything that shouldn't be there and devour-
> ing it.

Sue also drew strength from books on getting well and contacted
the Bristol Cancer Centre for advice on vitamin therapy.
Meanwhile she had written to me and in April 1994 she had her
first healing session. Shortly afterwards she started a course of
radiotherapy. This eventually affected her windpipe and her
ability to swallow food.

> I visited Matthew during this difficult period. I hadn't
> been able to swallow food for a few days. I felt great heat
> when Matthew laid his hands on my chest. After the
> session I was terribly hungry and we stopped on the
> journey back. I tucked into a huge meal with gusto and
> had no problem at all. My ability to swallow had been
> restored – it was quite remarkable.

Like Carol, Sue was determined that her life should not be ruled
by her cancer and she developed a healthy disregard for some of
the medical advice she was given. When to everybody's surprise
a chemotherapy match was found for her condition, Sue wanted
to try it even though the consultant could make no promises that
it would work. Sue said, 'I was thrilled, over the moon.' She was
advised not to socialize while she underwent chemotherapy
because her immune system would be suppressed and this
would make her particularly susceptible to opportunistic infec-
tions. She went out almost every night and did not get so much
as a sniffle. Her view on this was:

> I can only think it was the healing with Matthew and my
> visualizations that kept me so well through it all . . . The
> first year came and went. My consultant was so pleased
> that I was still still alive and so well, he jokingly said, 'keep
> on proving me wrong'.

Sue is a shining example of someone who has not passively
stood by and let others plan a health strategy for her. She has
made her own decisions and taken control of her illness. After
that first year she decided to keep coming to me once a month
until she felt she had no further need of it. She lessened the frequency of her visualizations with my *Women with Cancer* tape,
which she had begun to use at the outset of the chemotherapy.
She felt that 'things had changed inside' and returned to the
Fighting Back tape, which she describes as 'much gentler. I saw
myself well and growing old in the years to come'.

At the time of writing, Sue is clear of cancer and fighting fit.
She is still taking her vitamins, and watching her diet. Her consultant has told her to just keep doing what she has been doing.
He and his team have been 'wonderfully supportive and very
open to alternative therapies and healing. Of course I was glad
to have conventional treatment when it was offered. If one wants
to live then my advice would be to try everything possible.'

* * *

Healing does not cure every ill and when I began to give Gig
treatment – shortly after the appearance of the mystery lesion –
I could no more guarantee her a successful outcome – on
whatever level that might take place – than I could any of my
other patients. Healing is set up in such a way, it seems, that it
is difficult for the healer to fall victim to hubris, and works to a
design which cannot be manipulated.

My efforts intensified once cancer was diagnosed. I gave her
healing every day until she began to experience the side-effects
of the radiotherapy treatment. From this point on I left it to her

to decide when she would like to receive it. In the beginning I
felt very self-conscious and inhibited. I was reminded of how I
used to feel when I first gave healing and had not learned to
dissociate myself emotionally. It can be difficult to make the distinction between emotional detachment and the empathy and
compassion that every healer must bring to his work. Many
novice healers find themselves experiencing the pain and distress
of the people they are trying to heal because they have not
achieved this separation.

Kitaro's music helped me to solve the problem with Gig. One
day when I was giving her healing, I turned up the volume on
the CD player to the point where the speakers were visibly vibrat-
ing, obliterating all thoughts and inhibitions. That did the trick.
Thankfully, it was not necessary to play the music at a deafening
level on subsequent occasions.

There are degrees of being in the right state for giving healing.
I cannot always 'fly' and experience the ultimate. When I do, it
is like reaching the edge of one cosmos and finding gates
opening on to another. I am filled with a joy that must be akin
to what some mystics have described as 'ecstasy'. In this state I
am aware of the complete connectedness of all beings. There
are no barriers, no differences, no judgements.

On the numerous occasions I have reached this ecstatic state,
I have seen a figure. He has the build and look of a gigantic
Sumo wrestler, although one that is stark naked, covered with
hair and – perhaps rather incongruously – exudes joy, love and
freedom. He came as a blinding vision on the first occasion, exe-
cuting back flips, somersaults and other amazing acrobatics. I
wondered how anyone so fat and unathletic could perform such
movements. He said, as if to answer my unspoken question, 'The
only reason I am so fat is because I am so full of love.' He does
not always speak, and when he does he limits himself to one,
usually cryptic, phrase.

The figure appeared once when I was giving Gig healing. It
was during her rest period between the five weeks of combined
chemotherapy and radiotherapy and the final two weeks of

radiotherapy. I was playing Kitaro's music – I usually am when
he appears – and became aware of him almost immediately. He
was doing the most extraordinary dance with what looked like
a Samurai sword, hurling it around and spinning it on his finger.
I heard him say, 'When you are strong you don't need the sword.'
Afterwards I wondered whether the session had been different in
any way for Gig. Without my asking, she told me that she
thought the tumour had gone.

A week later we went back to the Hammersmith for Gig to
have an X-ray and examination before she started her final two
weeks of treatment. Neither revealed any sign of the tumour.
The doctors were pleased that it seemed to have disappeared
faster than they had anticipated. Gig and I were delighted.
However, it was recommended that the treatment plan should
be followed and that the further two weeks of radiotherapy
should be administered, just to be on the safe side. We went
home confident that the combination of therapies was working.

* * *

We can pride ourselves on being understanding and compas-
sionate, but none of us knows what someone else is going
through until, filled with fear and confusion, we have groped
our way to the end of that same tunnel. When Sue Wallis first
wrote to me she commented in her letter that she hoped that
she was 'more than just a victim, a tumour'. She is immeasur-
ably more. Some people only discover their real worth or an
appreciation of themselves through a brush with adversity. Such
an experience undoubtedly concentrates the mind, focusing it
minutely on the aspects of life that are important.

Sharing our feelings and giving of ourselves honestly are
especially important at such times. One refrain which has
cropped up repeatedly in my workshops over the years is, 'If
only' – 'If only I had said . . .', 'If only I had had time to . . .', 'If
only I had been there'. In these circumstances healing is not only
about healing one person who has got a problem on a physical

level. It is also about healing the people around that individual, and maybe healing the way forward for them.

I am often asked which case has had the most impact on me. I would put the following at the top.

Chris was a very sporty, no-nonsense guy in his forties who had been diagnosed with cancer. I was not sure what I could do for him and at our first meeting, I said: 'Let me have three sessions with you. If nothing happens, I doubt that I can do any more.' He came on a monthly basis and by the last session it was obvious that his condition was deteriorating. Afterwards, he looked at me and said: 'So, that's my three sessions, is it? You're going to kick me out now, are you, because we're not getting anywhere?'

I was shocked and for the first time realized that my attitude must have come across to him – and probably others – as unfeeling. He said 'Let me tell you something. You might think that you're not doing anything. You know and I know that the cancer is getting worse, but what you may not know is when I leave you it is like walking out on air and I am completely pain-free for the next two weeks. That is all I am asking of you. Please, don't cast me aside. I may not survive, but it's quality of life to me that is important.'

Somewhat against expectation, Chris survived for a further six months. The last time he came to see me he looked absolutely dreadful and I knew that I had lost him. He was his usual honest self and I remember him saying, 'I know I've only got a few days left. Come on, hit me with it one more time!' After the healing session his wife was a little late in picking him up and we had time for a chat. We talked about what we learn from death and serious illness, and about their spiritual implications. I mentioned the 'if only' factor and how heavily it seemed to weigh on many bereaved people.

When Chris got up to leave, he hugged me. We both knew we would not see each other again. A couple of days later his wife telephoned the office and asked to speak to me. I knew what her message would be and expected her to sound flat and depressed. Not a bit of it. In the background I could hear loud music playing. She told me that Chris had died the day before. After they had left me and driven home, he had taken her into their living room, sat her down and told her that he was about to die. Before this acknowledgement, he had always been full of bravado and plans for the future. A keen yachtsman, he had told her about the races he was going to win and the competitions he was going to enter. She told me that she and her daughter had felt fraudulent because they knew he was not going to make it, but love and loyalty necessitated that they should keep up the charade.

When Chris told her he was going to die, she felt as though a great weight had been lifted from her shoulders. Suddenly, they could be open and honest with each other again. They spent most of the next twenty-four hours looking through their photograph albums and as they did so reminisced about the great shared events in their life: marriage, the birth of their daughter, wonderful holidays and all the other happy occasions. They also held each other and forgave each other for the times when perhaps inadvertently they had caused each other pain or unhappiness. In the last hours of Chris's life they reached the point where there was no unfinished business. Everything of importance to either of them had been discussed and resolved.

At the end of our conversation, his wife said, 'I cannot thank you enough for that. I cannot tell you how much I will grieve for him and miss him. But although Chris has gone, for me the healing was actually in that we had time to say "Goodbye" and to say it properly.'

Chris had left behind some specific instructions for his funeral, she told me. He wanted all those attending to go with happy faces and smiles. He wanted his favourite soft rock music to be played and not the standard sombre funereal fare. When she said this, I realized that soft rock was what I could hear playing in the background. His last instruction had thrown the undertaker into confusion – his body was to be placed in a coffin painted white with blue 'go-fast' stripes (the motif on his racing yacht) down the sides so that when he was brought into the church all his friends could have one last laugh with him. He wanted to take his leave on a positive note and be remembered in that light.

Life and death leave a legacy. Each of us can choose what ours will be. To my way of thinking, Chris got it absolutely right. That is not to say that his friends and family would not shed many tears at his loss or that he would not be missed, but through his actions he freed them. So often the past holds us back. To borrow a saying from Ram Dass, each of us has to be here now. For me, Gig's recent illness has confirmed the wisdom of valuing each day as it comes. If you live for the moment, you tend not to take so much for granted, and this enables you to experience a far wider range of joys. I am easier to please in this respect than I used to be. I derive intense pleasure from simple things, such as the shape of a flower. I am not so much a couch potato as a home potato, who is more than content to sit in his garden listening to the bird-song.

My only addiction now is to Scrabble, a state of affairs for which Gig is entirely to blame. She was a really good player when we met and used to beat me mercilessly. Once my competitive tendency got over the shock and humiliation, it devised a strategy for redressing the balance. Now every match is close-run and we take it in turns to crow.

Our families and friends are bemused by this shared passion. The garden they can understand, but what sort of people insist on taking a Scrabble board wherever they go, even on holiday? It was handy in Grenada, where it rained all day and gave us a legitimate excuse for playing from eight in the morning until midnight. Clear blue skies did not stop play on Barbados. My parents came out for a few days while we were there and stayed in the same hotel. My father was completely nonplussed and not a little irritated when we spent much of the time sitting under a palm tree, playing. He is a very restless, inquisitive man, who has to be 'doing'.

Tranquillity seems to suit me and I would like the second

half of my life to be less eventful than the first. I suppose I shall have to continue to accept that quirky happenings will still occur. The energetic poltergeist of my youth is no longer in evidence, but from time to time the inexplicable still occurs.

In 1998 my assistants, Jane and Pat, and I stopped work a couple of days short of the start of the official Christmas holiday. On that last day we called a halt at four in the afternoon and Jane and Pat came into the kitchen to wish us all Happy Christmas before starting their break. I had the car keys in my hand as I planned to leave immediately for Bury St Edmunds with Gig and the children to do the food shopping for the Christmas festivities.

I put the keys on the corner of the dresser as I went towards Jane and Pat to give them each a hug. I could still see the keys as I was hugging Jane. When I turned to pick them up a few moments later, they had vanished. We turned the kitchen upside down trying to find them, and every other room in the house I had been in during the course of the day. In the end, we had to admit defeat and use the spare set.

We drove into the centre of Bury St Edmunds and found a parking space outside the first of the several food shops we were to visit. By the end of the afternoon the large boot was full of groceries, drink and our Christmas turkey and we were looking forward to having the pizza we had promised the children in return for helping with our shopping marathon.

Before leaving the car for the final time, near the restaurant, I went round to check the boot. I would not normally do this, and would trust the central locking to work as it should, but I was very aware of the value of the contents and needed to satisfy myself that the shopping we had amassed would still be there when we got back. When I reached the rear of the car, I found the missing set of keys dangling in the lock.

Equally mystifying was what happened after Gig and I had taken Henrietta back to school at the start of her spring term at Oakham in January 1999. We were not far from home, driving through the village of Horringer. We go through this place regularly and take for granted the fact that nearby Ickworth House had been home to the Marquesses of Bristol for generations.

For no reason Gig and I started talking about the Marquess and wondering how he was. We had seen him once in a local restaurant and had remarked on how ill he looked. Gig wondered what would happen to his title when he died, and who it would pass to, as he had no heirs. Neither of us knew the answer to that and the conversation ended. Later that evening we were watching television when suddenly, without any intervention from either Gig or I, the set switched from the programme we were watching to Teletext, which was announcing the death of the Marquess of Bristol.

There is no way the television could have changed channels without the use of the remote-control hand set, and that device had been several feet away from both Gig and me when the switch occurred.

I do not find healing energy as difficult to explain as the energies involved in these two stories. I regard healing energy as an unconditional universal force for good. Many people may find it difficult to believe in something whose existence cannot be proved scientifically. I wonder how many people would be prepared to say they could not believe in love because it has not been conclusively measured and quantified by science. Most people – even people who may be sceptical about the existence of healing energy – believe in love. I suspect that they believe in it for the same reason that I believe in healing energy, because they have felt its effects, as a child, parent, lover or friend. We measure love by the effect it has on our lives. We should treat healing energy in the same way.

I suppose every human being spends the entirety of the life granted him trying to get to the bottom of who he is and why he is here. People who have an obvious vocation are always regarded as being immensely fortunate by those who do not. A talent or ability is often seen to provide a justification for an individual's existence and elevate that individual above the rest. That seems to miss the point about life.

It is what we are as human beings that counts. In my case, merely possessing a gift imbued with heavy spiritual overtones does not make me a better person or my life choices easier. It is also debatable whether those we elevate are solely responsible for their gifts. Take healing. Wherever the energy that I use comes from, it is not from me directly. I believe it comes from without and works through me. I am merely someone who has managed to use effectively what he has been given. I am simply doing my job.

Many discoveries have been made on a hunch, an intuition, or have taken shape during dream states. One wonders where the inspiration for these comes from. Professor Brian Josephson once told me that most of his discoveries, including the one that won him the Nobel Prize, had come to him while he was meditating. The difficulty for him was that having picked up the answer, he then had to work backwards from the solution to show how he had arrived at it. This suggests that knowledge of which we are as yet ignorant is somehow already in the ether, waiting to be plucked out and used. It raises interesting questions about the nature of creativity. Does it originate within the individual or is the creative person tapping into some source beyond himself?

During the time I practised automatic drawing, I doubted that the spirit of the artist whose work those drawings most closely resembled was responsible for producing them. It did not seem feasible that Dürer, Picasso or Goya would be hanging around for years – in Dürer's case, 450 – after his physical death and continuing to churn out similar drawings through a schoolboy. Life after death must surely hold more than that. It may be that every act of creation or thought generates an energy that is never lost and in particular circumstances – such as a meditative state – may be accessed later.

When I used to practise absent healing, on several occasions someone would call and thank me profusely for some miraculous recovery they said had occurred in a relative or friend after I had been asked to give healing to that person. We would find no trace of the letter or the individual referred to when we went through our records to make a note of this occurrence in the appropriate file. A day or two later the letter would arrive. In these cases healing occurred before we knew of the need for it.

I have spent many hours trying to draw conclusions from such events and understand what, or who, is making the healing work. Is it the person writing the letter? Is it some unconscious connection with me? Is the intent sufficient to make healing work, perhaps through the intervention of some higher force? Are requests for help, for example, really prayers that are picked up and answered by that force? These and similar imponderables have helped me to put my own contribution to healing in a broader context.

I rather like Steven Levine's idea of healing as a state of being. It is not an act. There are people who exude a wonderful quality – energy, aura, call it what you will. You have only to be around them a short while and you feel recharged, revitalized. They are life's natural healers. Equally, there are others who seem to have the effect of sucking the life force out of you after a very short time in their company. The people in this second category are invariably negative, full of moans and incapable of seeing the good in anything, even goodness itself. That state of being is the antithesis of healing, of what – for want of a better word – I call spirituality.

My definition of spirituality owes nothing to the belief systems of the established Churches. I am as proudly irreligious now as I was in my childhood. Being spiritual and being religious can be – and often are – separate ways of life. Too many religious people regard faith as an insurance policy, covering them against the wrath of that unknown Almighty. Spirituality is a code for living.

Many of the people who come to my workshops are looking to healing to fill a spiritual vacuum. Maybe my perception is distorted because the people I see tend not to be respecters of orthodoxy in any of its forms, but I believe that many people nowadays are questioning of anything that is establishment, whether in the area of science, religion or politics. Science was once a god for many people. Now it has been found to have feet of clay, and people realize it does not have all the answers. Orthodox religion, too, has seen an erosion in its influence, and many of those who are searching for a meaning to life are looking elsewhere for the answer.

People like myself are in a way bridging the divide that has opened up. We seem to be reaching a coming of age, certainly where religion is concerned. People want to 'do it for themselves', but they still want a few ground rules. Because I am a healer, they assume that I am able to provide them. I am in the same situation as every other mortal in that I do not know what life will throw at me next.

One thing my experiences have convinced me of is that there is a purpose to life and it is not just a bad joke being played on us by some all-powerful force we cannot know. I believe we choose our lives and that we may choose many different lives in order to learn the lessons we need to learn. It is through this learning process that we grow and evolve on a spiritual level. Soul-wise I think we are migratory and we tend to move in groupings. We and the other souls making up the group are like a dandelion clock that has been blown on, scattering us so we replant in a different part of the universe and yet are within reach of one another in our various lives. We may reconnect as lovers, spouses, friends, parents, children.

Everything that happens to us in life is potentially an opportunity for growth, but each of us has a choice as to how we deal with the opportunities presented to us. Some years ago I received a letter from the mother of a severely handicapped child I had been treating who died. This boy had been incapable of doing anything for himself and had relied almost solely on his parents and brother and sister for his physical welfare. His mother wrote that after his death many people, including relatives, had commented on how terrible life must be for them, first with the burden of the child's disability and latterly with his death. Her perspective was totally different from their perception of what it must be. Those people, she said, did not realize how the family had grown through their shared experience and that the child had given them all a great gift.

Sometimes healing does not work because in a spiritual context it is not the right time for it to work. It might be that someone is learning in some way or evolving from an experience of illness. The person who has died might have gone as far as he or she can in this life, and it is time for them to become 'homeless' and leave that particular identity, or it might be that other people around them are meant to learn from the experience.

If each of us could take from each experience and look at it positively, as something to be learned from and cherished, life would become inseparable from meaning. We could not be swallowed up by the many black holes in our consciousness. Albert Einstein once remarked that the world was 'becoming a dangerous place, not because of the bad things people do but because of those who just watch and do nothing.'

By being positive, adjusting our consciousness so we always look for the good in other people and to a higher purpose, we can make the world a better, safer place. We may not think it can make any difference but when that sort of action is taken by millions of lives, it cannot fail to have a beneficial effect. The way we think conditions our actions. Our thoughts give the world its spiritual energy. If those thoughts are negative the energy they generate is liable to be destructive. When I demonstrate healing, it is not necessarily just the person I am working with one-to-one who gets the benefit. Healing has a ripple effect, and the positive energy channelled at the centre flows out to the edges. When we learn to live as positive beings we are enabling ourselves to have at least one foot in the stars.

*   *   *

Wendy Rayner was one of the few people who stepped over the line that separates my friends from my patients. Wendy had breast cancer that went into her bones and eventually into her liver and brain. She came to me as a patient and by the time of her death was much loved by both Gig and I. She was drawn to the area of Suffolk where Gig and I live, and bought a cottage up on the hill near us. Our friendship was characterized by endless talks about life and death over good food and wine. The philosophy we shared is encapsulated by a piece of writing which Wendy wanted to be read at her funeral. It is called 'Risks'.

To laugh is to risk appearing a fool.

To weep is to risk appearing sentimental.

To reach out for another is to risk involvement.

To expose feelings is to risk exposing your true self.

To place your ideas, your dreams before the crowd is to risk their loss.

To love is to risk not being loved in return.

To live is to risk dying.

To hope is to risk despair.

To try is to risk failure.

But risks must be taken because the greatest hazard in life is to risk nothing. The person who risks nothing does nothing, has nothing, is nothing. He may avoid suffering and sorrow, but he simply cannot learn, feel, change, grow, love, live. Chained by his certitudes, he is a slave: he has forfeited freedom.

Only a person who risks is free.

PIATKUS BOOKS

If you have enjoyed reading this book, you may be interested in other titles published by Piatkus. These include:

Teach Yourself to Meditate by Eric Harrison
Yesterday's Children by Jenny Cockell
Your Healing Power by Jack Angelo